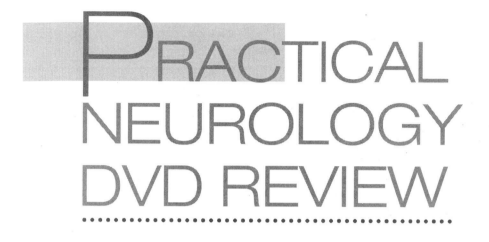

PRACTICAL NEUROLOGY DVD REVIEW

D0113497

PRACTICAL NEUROLOGY DVD REVIEW

■ BY JOSÉ BILLER, MD, FACP, FAAN, FAHA
Loyola University Chicago
Stritch School of Medicine
Department of Neurology
Maywood, Illinois

Contributions By
James D. Fleck, MD and Robert M. Pascuzzi, MD

Technical Assistance By
Rocky Rothrock and Denise Mehner

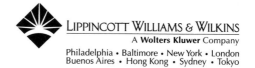

LIPPINCOTT WILLIAMS & WILKINS
A **Wolters Kluwer** Company
Philadelphia • Baltimore • New York • London
Buenos Aires • Hong Kong • Sydney • Tokyo

Acquisitions Editor: Anne M. Sydor
Developmental Editor: Nicole Dernosky
Project Manager: David Murphy
Senior Manufacturing Manager: Ben Rivera
Marketing Manager: Adam Glazer
Production Services: TechBooks
Printer: Edwards Brothers

Care has been taken to confirm the accuracy of the information presented and to describe
generally accepted practices. However, the authors, editors, and publisher are not responsible for errors or omissions or for any consequences from application of the information in
this book and make no warranty, expressed or implied, with respect to the currency, com-
pleteness, or accuracy of the contents of the publication. Application of this information in
a particular situation remains the professional responsibility of the practitioner.
The authors, editors, and publisher have exerted every effort to ensure that drug selection and
dosage set forth in this text are in accordance with current recommendations and practice
at the time of publication. However, in view of ongoing research, changes in government
regulations, and the constant flow of information relating to drug therapy and drug reactions,
the reader is urged to check the package insert for each drug for any change in indications
and dosage and for added warnings and precautions. This is particularly important when
the recommended agent is a new or infrequently employed drug.
Some drugs and medical devices presented in this publication have Food and Drug Administration (FDA) clearance for limited use in restricted research settings. It is the responsibility
of the health care provider to ascertain the FDA status of each drug or device planned for
use in their clinical practice.

10 9 8 7 6 5 4 3 2 1

To the memory of my beloved wife Célika T. Biller (1949–2003)

As virtuous men passe mildly away,
    And whisper to their soules, to goe,
Whilst some of their sad friends doe say,
    The breath goes now, and some say, no:

So let us melt, and make no noise,
    No teare-floods, nor sigh-tempests move,
T'were prophanation of our joyes
    To tell the layetie our love.

Moving of th'earth brings harmes and feares,
    Men reckon what it did and meant,
But trepidation of the spheares,
    Though greater farre, is innocent.

Dull sublunary lovers love
    (Whose soule is sense) cannot admit
Absence, because it doth remove
    Those things which elemented it.

But we by a love, so much refin'd,
    That our selves know not what it is,
Inter-assured of the mind,
    Care lesse, eyes, lips, and hands to misse.

Our two soules therefore, which are one,
    Though I must goe, endure not yet
A breach, but an expansion,
    Like gold to ayery thinesse beate.

If they be two, they are two so
    As stiffe twin compasses are two,
Thy soule the fixt foot, makes no show
    To move, but doth, if th'other doe.

And though it in the center sit,
    Yet when the other far doth rome,
It leanes, and hearkens after it,
    And growes erect, as that comes home.

Such wilt thou be to mee, who must
    Like th'other foot, obliquely runne;
Thy firmnes drawes my circle just,
    And makes me end, where I begunne.

(John Donne [1572–1631], *A Valediction: Forbidding Mourning*)

CONTENTS

■ SECTION 5: EXTRAPYRAMIDAL 85

■ SECTION 9: NEUROINFECTIOUS 139

■ SECTION 10: NEUROOTOLOGY 143

■ SECTION 11: NUTRITIONAL/METABOLIC 149

■ SECTION 12: HEADACHES/PAIN 153

CONTRIBUTING AUTHORS

José Biller, MD, FACP, FAAN, FAHA
Loyola University Chicago
Stritch School of Medicine
Department of Neurology
Maywood, Illinois

James D. Fleck, MD
Indiana University School of Medicine
Indianapolis, Indiana

Robert M. Pascuzzi, MD
Indiana University School of Medicine
Indianapolis, Indiana

Rocky Rothrock
Photographer
Office of Visual Media
Indiana University School of Medicine

Denise Mehner
Indiana University School of Medicine
Indianapolis, Indiana

"We see what we look for."
"You can observe a lot by watching."—Yogi Berra

Neurologic problems are common in general medical practice and often are a heavy burden for patients and their families. Practitioners, residents/fellows in training, and medical students encounter these disorders with increasing frequency because of the growing size of the aging population.

Current assessment formats for residents/fellows and medical students' education underemphasize bedside teaching. Faculty members often do not observe trainees performing physical examinations during their training.

This educational material offers new venues for teaching and learning the essentials of neurology by utilizing an interactive patient based (real-world situation) audiovisual electronic format (incorporating key semiological, neuroimaging, or other ancillary data when appropriate). One hundred and two carefully edited video clips of patients with an array of commonly and unusually encountered neurological problems are used to teach the following fundamental principles of bedside neurology: (1) description and localization of findings, (2) differential diagnosis, (3) evaluation, (4) management, and (5) counseling. The first two items are considered essential aspects of knowledge, while the last three represent more advanced knowledge and skills. The cases range from the very easy to the very challenging in order to meet the needs of all segments of the intended audience. Each clinical vignette is accompanied by a balanced, practical, and non-encyclopedic written discussion that includes basic learning objectives, an executive summary, and recommended reading material.

This audiovisual electronic teaching format may be somewhat unorthodox. However, it is actually more effective in its approach because the technology lends itself to displaying the skills necessary for a physician to form a patient's neurological diagnosis, which is largely based on an effective history, interpersonal communication, and visual information. Therefore, it may help to clarify at the outset what this material does and does not set out to accomplish: It is not meant to be an encyclopedic audiovisual electronic clinical neurology library. It is an interactive tool for learning/teaching relevant and practical neurology problems, narrated by real patients—not by actors or "simulated patients," as is the trend in current medical education.

Two hundred and sixty multiple choice questions, with cross-references to the video clips and to the second edition of *Practical Neurology,* when pertinent, are included.

On completion of this program, users will be able to recognize an improvement in their core knowledge of:

- Neurological examination and techniques
- Clinical reasoning
- Abstract problem solving
- Attentiveness
- Critical curiosity
- Evidence-based neurology

I hope this educational material brings the highest-quality neurological care to as many patients as possible and encourages medical students and residents/fellows to elect careers in academic neurology.

José Biller, MD, FACP, FAAN, FAHA

ACKNOWLEDGMENT

I am forever indebted to each of my patients for enthusiastically agreeing to participate in this project. The editing and final production of this material are the result of the efforts of a dedicated and highly talented and professional team. I especially thank Rocky Rothrock, for the countless hours of passionate video editing; Denise Mehner, from the Office of Visual Media at Indiana University School of Medicine; Anne Sydor, from Lippincott Williams & Wilkins, for her constant encouragement; Nicole Dernoski, from Lippincott Williams & Wilkins, for her editorial efforts and professionalism; Phyllis Cowherd and MaryAnn Baumhart, for their extraordinary patience in the production of this material and for their wonderful secretarial and administrative support; my colleagues at Indiana University and Loyola University; and of course my children, Sofia, Gabriel, and Rebecca for their constant support.

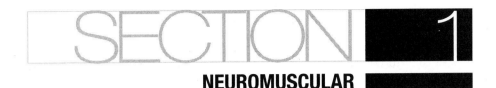

SECTION 1

NEUROMUSCULAR

CASE 1

BILATERAL CARPAL TUNNEL IN PREGNANCY

OBJECTIVES

- To name the nerve affected in carpal tunnel syndrome.
- To name the most common symptoms of carpal tunnel syndrome.
- To name the most useful diagnostic test to confirm carpal tunnel syndrome.
- To name the most common treatments for carpal tunnel syndrome.

VIGNETTE

A 32-year-old woman, G1, P0, 38-week gestation, complained of bilateral hand numbness and pain for the last 2 weeks.

CASE SUMMARY

Median neuropathy at the wrist (carpal tunnel syndrome) is the most common entrapment neuropathy. The median nerve is entrapped at the carpal tunnel of the wrist, which is made up on the sides and floor by carpal bones and on the roof by the transverse carpal ligament. The most common symptoms are wrist, hand, and arm pain associated with paresthesias in the hand. The pain typically is worse at night, disturbing sleep. The paresthesias are most frequently present in the thumb, index, middle, and lateral aspect of the ring finger. Symptoms may be noted with such activities as driving or holding a phone and can also be noted during pregnancy as in our patient. The incidence of preeclampsia in pregnant patients with carpal tunnel syndrome ranges between 9% and 20%.

Paresthesias may be elicited by gentle tapping over the median nerve (Tinel's sign) or by having the patient hold her wrist in a flexed position (Phalen's maneuver).

Weakness of the median innervated muscles, especially the abductor pollicis brevis (APB), may be present. Atrophy of the thenar eminence may be noted in more severe cases. Nerve conduction studies and electromyography (EMG) are the most useful tests to confirm the diagnosis. The most common treatments include removal of provoking factors and a neutral wrist splint. If unsuccessful, surgical decompression is the most definitive treatment. The role of steroid injections is controversial.

■ SELECTED REFERENCES

Biller J, ed. *Practical neurology,* 2nd ed. Philadelphia: Lippincott Williams & Wilkins, 2002:Chapter 24.
Ekman-Orderberg G, Sageback S, Orderberg G. Carpal tunnel syndrome in pregnancy. *Acta Obstet Gynecol Scand* 1987;66:233–235.

■ SEE QUESTIONS: 3, 16, 17, 57, 79

CASE 2

ULNAR NEUROPATHY AT THE ELBOW

OBJECTIVES

- To name the most common symptoms of an ulnar neuropathy.
- To name the most useful diagnostic test to confirm an ulnar neuropathy.
- To name the most common site of ulnar neuropathy.
- To name the most common treatments for ulnar neuropathy.

VIGNETTE

Following a bilateral hernia operation, this 70-year-old man complained of paresthesias on the fourth and fifth digits of his left hand. He also noticed some decrease in grip strength of that hand.

CASE SUMMARY

The ulnar nerve can be compressed at a variety of sites along its course from the brachial plexus to the hand. By far the most common site of compression is at the elbow where the nerve passes through a fibroosseous canal called the cubital tunnel. The most common sensory symptoms are numbness and paresthesias of the medial forearm, medial hand, fifth digit, and medial half of the fourth digit. Motor symptoms most commonly are weakness of hand muscles or decreased hand dexterity. Atrophy of the hypothenar eminence or first dorsal interosseous muscle may be noted. Electromyography (EMG) and nerve conduction studies are the most useful tests to confirm the diagnosis.

Conservative treatments such as avoidance of repetitive elbow flexion and extension and avoidance of direct pressure on the elbow, perhaps adding elbow protectors, are used first. Surgical options can be explored if conservative measures fail. As in our patient, ulnar neuropathies have been associated with surgical procedures and general anesthesia. It appears to be more common in men and those with certain medical conditions. Diabetes is a frequent predisposing factor. Controversy exists as to the importance of patient positioning during surgery as a cause of perioperative ulnar neuropathy.

■ SELECTED REFERENCES

Biller J, ed. *Practical neurology,* 2nd ed. Philadelphia: Lippincott Williams & Wilkins, 2002:Chapter 24.
Dellon AL, Hament W, Gittelshon A. Non-operative management of cubital tunnels syndrome: an 8-year-prospective study. *Neurology* 1993;43:1673–1677.

■ SEE QUESTIONS: 3, 4, 16, 57, 80, 81

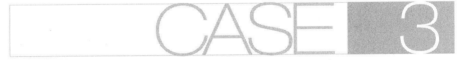

PERIPHERAL FACIAL NERVE PALSY

OBJECTIVES

▨ To name the most common symptoms of facial nerve palsy.
▨ To name the distinguishing characteristics of an upper motor neuron and a lower motor neuron facial weakness.
▨ To name some common causes of facial nerve palsy.
▨ To name the most common treatments for Bell's palsy.

VIGNETTE

A 65-year-old man with a history of carcinoid tumor had new onset of left facial weakness.

CASE SUMMARY

The facial nerve is a mixed motor-sensory and parasympathetic nerve supplying the muscles of facial expression, mucous membranes of the oral and nasal cavities, and salivary and lacrimal glands. It also conveys taste sensation from the anterior two-thirds of the tongue via the lingual nerve and chorda tympani. Facial weakness is the most common symptom of a facial nerve palsy. Aching of the ear or mastoid region may be present. Patients may complain of numbness or an unusual sensation of the face, but sensory testing should be normal. Taste may be impaired if the lesion is proximal to the chorda tympani. Sounds may be exaggerated (hyperacusis) if a lesion is proximal to the nerve branch supplying the stapedius muscle, which typically helps dampen loud sounds.

Our patient had a Bell's palsy. Bell's palsy is more common in adults, patients with diabetes, and pregnant women. Herpes simplex virus has been suspected as an inciting factor. A short course of corticosteroids and oral antiviral agents is advocated by some authors. Artificial tears during the day and lubricating ophthalmic ointment at night are recommended to prevent the complications of corneal exposure.

■ SELECTED REFERENCES

Adour KK, Ruboyianes JM, Von Doerstein PG, et al. Bell's palsy treatment with acyclovir and prednisone compared with prednisone alone: a double-blind, randomized, controlled trial. *Ann Otol Rhinol Laryngol* 1996;105:371–378.

Biller J, ed. *Practical neurology,* 2nd ed. Philadelphia: Lippincott Williams & Wilkins, 2002:Chapter 15.

■ SEE QUESTIONS: 84, 152, 153, 173, 190, 197, 235, 250

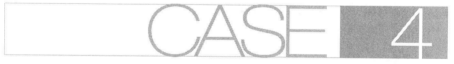

HYPOGLOSSAL NERVE PALSY

OBJECTIVES

▓ To name the location of the hypoglossal nucleus.
▓ To name the most common signs and symptoms of hypoglossal nerve palsy.
▓ To name the most common causes of hypoglossal nerve palsy.

VIGNETTE

A 60-year-old woman developed new onset vertex headache radiating to the left orbital region, left auricular region, left retromandibular area, and left posterior neck. She also had trouble chewing, swallowing, and controlling her tongue.

CASE SUMMARY

The hypoglossal nerve (CN XII) provides motor innervation to the intrinsic and extrinsic muscles of the tongue. The hypoglossal nucleus is located in the dorsomedial medulla. The hypoglossal nerve exits the skull through the hypoglossal canal located just above the foramen magnum. Its course is divided into the following segments: medullary, cisternal, skull base, nasopharyngeal and oropharyngeal, carotid space, and sublingual. A unilateral lesion, as in this patient, often leads to symptoms of trouble controlling the tongue when chewing, speaking, or perhaps swallowing. Examination of a unilateral lesion will show deviation of the tongue to the affected side as contralateral tongue protrusion is weakly opposed or unopposed.

There may also be ipsilateral tongue atrophy and fasciculations. Isolated CN XII palsy is an uncommon clinical presentation. Supranuclear CN XII lesions do not result in denervation atrophy of the tongue musculature as seen in our patient. The most common cause of unilateral hypoglossal nerve palsy is tumors. They can also be seen in multiple sclerosis, Guillain-Barré syndrome, trauma, stroke, surgery, and infections. T2-weighted magnetic resonance imaging (MRI) demonstrated asymmetric high-signal intensity on the left CN XII.

■ SELECTED REFERENCES

Badion MLS, Lim CCT, Teo J, et al. Solitary fibrous tumor of the hypoglossal nerve. *AJNR* 2003;24:343–345.
Keane JR. Twelfth nerve palsy. Analysis of 100 cases. *Arch Neurol* 1996;53:561–566.

■ SEE QUESTIONS: 84, 138, 235

CASE 5

BRACHIAL PLEXOPATHY (PARSONAGE-TURNER SYNDROME)

OBJECTIVES

▨ To review pertinent applied anatomy of the brachial plexus.
▨ To analyze most common etiologies of brachial plexopathies.
▨ To review current ancillary evaluation techniques of brachial plexus lesions.
▨ To briefly discuss clinical presentation and prognosis of idiopathic brachial plexitis (Parsonage-Turner syndrome).

VIGNETTE

A 53-year-old man complained of left neck and shoulder pain and arm weakness.

CASE SUMMARY

Evaluation and management of brachial plexopathies requires a thorough knowledge of neuroanatomy. The brachial plexus is formed from the ventral primary rami (spinal nerves or roots) of C-5 through T-1. A prefixed plexus (when C-4 contributes a branch to the brachial plexus) is seen in approximately two-thirds of cases. The brachial plexus is divided into five major components: (i) roots, (ii) trunks (upper, middle, and lower), (iii) divisions (anterior and posterior), (iv) cords (lateral, posterior, and medial), and (v) branches. Typically, the brachial plexus is composed of five roots, three trunks, six divisions (two for each trunk), and three cords (Fig. 5.1).

Brachial plexus injuries may be complete or incomplete. Injuries may be classified as preganglionic (proximal to the spinal ganglion) or postganglionic. Plexus injuries can result in muscle weakness, neck and shoulder pain, paresthesias or dysesthesias, absent muscle stretch reflexes, and sensory loss. Despite some clinical variations,

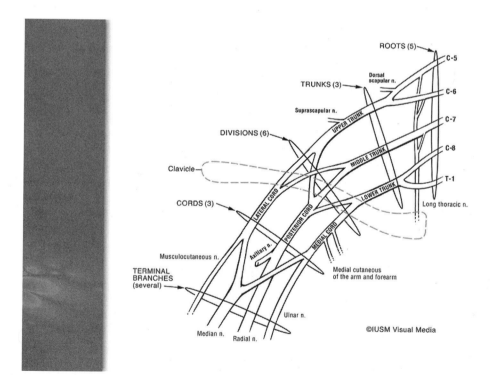

Figure 5.1
Anatomical Drawing of the Brachial Plexus

application of full pressure sensation to the thumb evaluates the corresponding C-6 spinal nerve, median nerve, and lateral cord; application of deep pressure to the middle finger evaluates the corresponding C-7 spinal nerve, median nerve, and lateral cord; whereas application of deep pressure to the little finger evaluates the corresponding C-8 spinal nerve, ulnar nerve, and the medial cord.

Motor signs are often more prominent than sensory changes in cases of plexopathy. Clinically relevant motor function to be tested should include shoulder abduction (C-5); elbow flexion, forearm pronation and supination (C-6); extensors of the forearm, hand, and fingers (C-7); finger extensors, finger flexors, and wrist flexors (C-8); and hand intrinsics (T-1).

In our patient, the motor signs involved predominantly the deltoid, biceps, brachioradialis, supraspinatus, and infraspinatus and were consistent with an upper plexus lesion. Sensation was intact. The biceps and brachioradialis reflexes were depressed on the involved side. High-energy trauma to the upper extremity and neck can cause a variety of lesions of the brachial plexus. Upper trunk brachial plexopathies (Erb-Duchenne type, C5-6) may result from traumatic separation of the head and shoulder, birth injury, and idiopathic brachial plexitis (neuralgic amyotrophy or Parsonage-Turner syndrome) as in our patient.

Parsonage-Turner syndrome (neuralgic amyotrophy) is an idiopathic brachial plexopathy most commonly seen in young adults and characterized by intense cervical and shoulder pain and shoulder girdle and upper extremity weakness and atrophy. Most cases are sporadic; a much rarer familial form occurs as an autosomal dominant variety.

The prognosis of patients with Parsonage-Turner syndrome is generally good, with a slow but progressive recovery over 6 to 18 months. Diagnosis can be substantiated by electrophysiologic testing and MRI of the brachial plexus.

MRI is a useful tool for the diagnosis of postganglionic brachial plexus lesions. MR imaging findings are normal in cases of Parsonage-Turner syndrome. Cervical disc herniation should be included in the differential diagnosis.

Lower brachial plexopathies (Dejerine-Klumpke, C8 and T1) often result from trauma, especially arm traction in the abducted position, or malignancies (Pancoast tumor). Lower trunk or medial cord involvement is among the most common peripheral nervous system complication of coronary artery bypass graft surgery.

■ SELECTED REFERENCES

Aminoff MJ, Olney RK, Parry GJ, et al. Relative utility of different electrophysiologic techniques in the evaluation of brachial plexopathies. *Neurology* 1989;39:1136–1137.

Bilbey JH, Lamond RG, Mattrey RT. MR imaging of disorders of the brachial plexus. *J Magn Reson Imaging* 1994;4(Jan-Feb):13–18.

■ SEE QUESTIONS: 4, 16, 79, 81, 82, 91, 119

CASE 6

POLYNEUROPATHY/SENSORY NEURONOPATHY

OBJECTIVES

- To review the differential diagnosis of progressive sensory neuronopathy.
- To list empirical treatment options for immune mediated peripheral neuropathy.
- To summarize treatment options for chronic neuropathic pain.

VIGNETTE

A 37-year-old woman began having problems with numbness, tingling, and weakness in her feet. The symptoms gradually progressed to the point where she became wheelchair bound. She also lost about 60 to 70 pounds.

CASE SUMMARY

This 37-year-old woman has a one-year history of progressive painful numbness and tingling, initially in the feet and legs and subsequently spreading into the hands and face. She has symmetrical distal sensory loss including profound deficits of position and vibratory sense. Muscle stretch reflexes are absent. She has a severe sensory ataxia and Romberg sign. Sural nerve biopsy demonstrated demyelination but no inflammation.

Causes of subacute/chronic sensory neuronopathy include remote effect of malignancy, Sjögren's syndrome, pyridoxine toxicity, vitamin B_{12} deficiency, toxicity from chemotherapy (cisplatin), and a viral or immune-mediated inflammatory sensory ganglionopathy. In addition, a significant number of patients have no identifiable explanation. In this patient there is a past history of psychiatric disease as well as dramatic weight loss prior to the onset of symptoms. The psychiatric history should raise the chances of a toxic exposure, as well as the chances for an underlying connective tissue disease such as systemic lupus erythematosus (SLE). Additionally, all young patients with severe neuropathy and psychiatric symptoms should be screened for porphyria.

This patient has been screened for these conditions with Anti-Hu serology, Anti-Ro (SSA) cytoplasmic antibodies and Anti-La (SSB) antibodies (for Sjögren's syndrome), cerebrospinal fluid (CSF) for elevated protein (as would be seen with a chronic immune mediated or inflammatory process), B_{12} studies, along with blood work and scans looking for occult systemic disease including malignancy. Even though no malignancy has been detected, the patient's history of cigarette smoking and the lack of objective evidence for inflammation leave us with the need to remain vigilant with regard to the possibility of malignancy. A positron emission tomography (PET) scan (perhaps the most sensitive single screening test for occult malignancy) has been ordered.

The patient's course has progressed such that she has constant intense neuropathic pain and is wheelchair bound owing to severe sensory ataxia. Therefore, she has been treated empirically for an immune-mediated neuropathy with prednisone and azathioprine with a marginal clinical response. Plasma exchange and intravenous immunoglobin (i.v. Ig) are additional reasonable treatment options, given the severity of the patient's symptoms.

Treatment of neuropathic pain is a major challenge in this patient. For chronic burning tingling dysesthesias (as experienced by our patient), tricyclic antidepressants remain first-line therapy. Amitriptyline or nortriptyline beginning at 25 mg qhs and gradually increasing as tolerated to 2 mg per kg qhs will provide significant benefit in at least half of patients so treated. Second-line therapy centers on anticonvulsant drugs; carbamazepine and gabapentin are the most often used. When other measures fail, a trial of mexiletine is worth considering, although the patient must be carefully evaluated for underlying cardiac disease given the drug's tendency to produce cardiac arrhythmia.

■ SELECTED REFERENCES

Barohn RJ. Approach to peripheral neuropathy and neuronopathy. *Semin Neurol* 1998;18:7–18.
Biller J, ed. *Practical neurology,* 2nd ed. Philadelphia: Lippincott Williams & Wilkins, 2002:Chapter 46.

■ SEE QUESTIONS: 73, 74, 75, 172, 173, 186, 214, 215, 228, 230, 241

CASE 7

L-5 RADICULOPATHY (DISC HERNIATION)

OBJECTIVES

- To review risk factors for lumbar disc herniations.
- To review the clinical presentation of lumbar radiculopathies.
- To discuss the most common etiologies of lumbar radiculopathy.
- To review the management of lumbar disc disease with sciatica.

VIGNETTE

A 31-year-old man developed left buttock and low back pain approximately 1 month ago. The patient noted that at times the pain was severe and limited his walking and his ability to sit. He had no numbness or weakness; however, he had limitation of movement of his left leg secondary to his pain. He described the pain as a tight feeling in his left buttock shooting down his leg and sometimes up his back when standing or when sitting for prolonged periods. Alleviating factors were sitting with his hip flexed and internally rotated. He also noted relief with Percocet that lasted approximately 3 to 4 hours but did not completely alleviate the pain. He had no loss of bowel or bladder function. He has taken naproxen and cyclobenzaprine in the past with no benefit. He also received acupuncture over the past month with no benefit.

CASE SUMMARY

Low back pain is extremely common, but only a fraction of patients experiencing low back pain during their lifetime have lumbar radiculopathy or sciatica as a consequence of root irritation or compression. Herniation of a lumbar intervertebral disc is one of the most common causes of root compression. The avascular biconcave intervertebral discs are located between successive vertebral bodies. The disc's annular structure is composed of an outer annulus fibrosus and an inner portion, the nucleus pulposus. Most lumbar disc herniations occur between the fourth and fifth lumbar or the fifth lumbar and first sacral interspaces. The spinal nerves exit the spinal canal through the foramina at each level. A disc herniation most frequently irritates the displaced nerve root. Most discs rupture in a posterolateral direction. The incidence of disc rupture is the same among men and women. The epidemiology of lumbar disc herniations has revealed cigarette smoking as a risk factor.

The distribution of the leg pain is dependent on the level of nerve root irritation or compression. Radicular or root pain results from inflammation of the nerve root, which has a characteristic burning or lancinating quality. The pain is generally accompanied by dermatomal sensory loss, paresthesias, or dysesthesias. A pain drawing can be very helpful in assessing the dermatomal distribution. Compression of a motor nerve results in weakness, and compression of a sensory nerve results in numbness. Often, accompanying numbness or tingling occurs with a distribution similar to the pain. On examination, a positive straight leg raising sign is almost always present. However, a crossed straight leg raising sign may be even more predictive of a lumbar disc herniation. The back may appear scoliotic. Gait is often abnormal. Muscle weakness may be revealed, particularly when walking on heels and toes.

Our patient had a classic presentation of a lesion affecting the L-5 root, including the complaint of lower back, buttock, lateral thigh, and anterolateral calf pain, with associated objective neurological findings of weakness of great toe and foot dorsiflexion (tibialis anterior and extensor hallucis longus) and dermatomal numbness of the lateral leg, dorsomedial foot, and great toe. With L-5 root lesions, both the patellar and Achilles reflexes are spared.

With lesions affecting the S-1 root, the pain generally involves the posterolateral thigh and calf, extending into the heel and lateral toes, and the sensory disturbances generally involve the posterior calf and lateral foot. S-1 radiculopathies may cause weakness affecting the gastrocnemius and toe flexors, and the Achilles reflex is depressed.

MRI is very sensitive in delineating lumbar disc herniations. Computed tomography (CT) myelography may be required in certain instances. Imaging studies must be reserved for cases in which positive findings have been documented. EMG may be a useful adjunct in selective cases. Almost all patients with sciatica and disk herniations deserve a trial of medical therapy with bed rest, antiinflammatory agents, analgesics, and muscle relaxants. Once the patient has recovered from the worst radicular pain, physical therapy can be instituted. Surgery must be considered among patients with severe and disabling sciatica, those with poor response to at least 4 weeks of conservative therapy, or in patients with neurologic deficits such as a foot drop or bladder or bowel disturbances.

■ SELECTED REFERENCES

Biller J, ed. *Practical neurology,* 2nd ed. Philadelphia: Lippincott Williams & Wilkins, 2002:Chapter 23.

Brazis PW, Masdeu JC, Biller J. *Localization in clinical neurology,* 4th ed. Philadelphia: Lippincott Williams & Wilkins, 2001.

Frymoyer JW, Pope MH, Clements JH, et al. Risk factors in low-back pain. An epidemiological survey. *J Bone Joint Surg Am* 1983;65(Feb):213–218.

Weber H. Lumbar disk herniation. A prospective study of prognostic factors including a controlled trial. Part 1. *J Oslo City Hosp* 1978;28 (Mar-Apr):33–64.

■ SEE QUESTIONS: 5, 56, 83

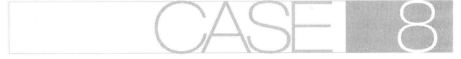

FOOT DROP: HISTORY OF ARTHROSCOPIC SURGERY

OBJECTIVES

▦ To review the clinical presentation of a lower motor neuron type of foot drop.
▦ To discuss the most common etiologies of foot drop.

VIGNETTE

A 61-year-old woman had a 2-week history of painless weakness of her right foot.

CASE SUMMARY

The common peroneal nerve descends into the leg as the lateral division of the sciatic nerve. The common peroneal nerve after rounding the head of the fibula divides into two branches: the deep peroneal (anterior tibial) nerve and the superficial peroneal nerve. Patients presenting with a foot drop often have lesions of either the peroneal nerve or L-5 spinal root. Neuropathy of the common peroneal nerve is a frequent clinical condition, generally caused by compression at the fibular head. Chronic compression from habitual leg crossing is a common mechanism. Peroneal entrapment neuropathy has also been reported from sitting in a cross-legged position (yoga foot drop), tibial fractures, casts, arthroscopic knee surgery, excessive climbing, nerve infarcts, Baker's cysts, hematoma, tumor, or leprosy.

Prolonged crash dieting may also result in peroneal neuropathy and foot drop. Compression of the peroneal nerve by an intraneural ganglion cyst or other masses (e.g., neurofibroma) may result in a painful foot drop. Bilateral foot drop may result from thiamine deficiency. Foot drop may also occur among pregnant patients who had a prolonged and difficult labor from compression of the lumbosacral trunk by a fetal head. Caustic effects on the sciatic nerve from certain drugs injected intramuscularly in the buttock, particularly among children, may result on a paralytic foot drop. Rarely, anterior compartmental syndromes affecting the deep division of the peroneal nerve present with similar manifestations.

Pressure palsy of the peroneal nerve at the fibular head results in foot drop and loss of sensation over the lateral calf, dorsal malleolus, and dorsum of the foot. Sensory loss is much more apparent with lesions of the superficial division of the peroneal nerve. With lesions of the deep division of the peroneal nerve, the sensory loss is often confined to a small area between the first and second toes. The weakness of ankle dorsiflexion, ankle eversion, and toe extension (dorsiflexion) is accompanied by an excessive slapping of the forefoot against the floor.

Palpation along the fibular head may elicit signs of tenderness or discover a mass. As demonstrated by our patient, with lesions at the fibular head, the deep branch of the peroneal nerve is affected more commonly than the whole nerve. Electrophysiological testing—nerve conduction velocities (NCVs) and EMG—are very helpful in the evaluation of these patients. MRI is also highly accurate in the evaluation of unusual causes of peroneal neuropathy.

■ SELECTED REFERENCES

Biller J, ed. *Practical neurology* 2nd ed. Philadelphia: Lippincott Williams & Wilkins, 2002:Chapter 25.

Brazis PW, Masdeu JC, Biller J. *Localization in clinical neurology,* 4th ed. Philadelphia: Lippincott Williams & Wilkins, 2001.

Nagel A, Greenebaum E, Singson RD, et al. Foot drop in a long-distance runner. An unusual presentation of neurofibromatosis. *Orthop Rev* 1994;23:526–530.

Vastamaki M. Decompression for peroneal nerve entrapment. *Acta Orthop Scand* 1986;57:551–554.

■ SEE QUESTIONS: 5, 56, 83

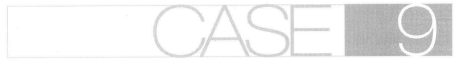

MOTOR NEURON DISEASE

OBJECTIVES

- To review the differential diagnosis of slowly progressive asymmetric lower extremity weakness.
- To list the diagnostic workup for patients with suspected motor neuron disease.
- To outline treatment strategies for patients with motor neuron disease.

VIGNETTE

A 34-year-old woman had a year-long history of right lower extremity weakness. Her problems began last November when she fell and twisted her ankle. Then in January of this year she noticed that she was walking in an unusual manner and was having difficulty raising her foot when walking. This became progressively worse and she has had frequent falls causing leg bruising. The patient had no speech or swallowing difficulties. She had no urinary or bowel complaints. She had no numbness or pain in her back or extremities. She had no upper extremity complaints.

CASE SUMMARY

The patient is a 34-year-old woman with 1 year of gradually progressive painless weakness and atrophy, initially affecting the right leg then spreading to the left, without sensory loss, bladder or bowel disturbance, back pain, or any nonmotor involvement. The examination demonstrates marked asymmetric lower extremity weakness of a lower motor neuron type without any upper motor neuron signs. Imaging of the spine, spinal fluid analysis, and routine laboratory studies are normal.

The electrophysiologic studies indicate relatively normal motor nerve conduction velocities, and the needle examination shows chronic and active neurogenic changes in multiple muscles. The localization appears to be that of weakness of a lower motor neuron type that includes anterior horn cell disease, polyradiculopathy of the lumbosacral segments, and peripheral motor neuropathy such as multifocal motor neuropathy. A myopathy is distinctly unlikely given the asymmetric as well as distal involvement in the lower extremities.

Motor neuron disease can begin in the leg or arm or bulbar muscles, and regardless of its initial presentation, over time slowly spreads at a steady pace. Although most patients have a course of amyotrophic lateral sclerosis (ALS) that runs 2 to 5 years, 20% of patients have a slower course longer than 5 years, and 10% longer than 10 years. The absence of upper motor neuron signs at this juncture makes it problematic to call this probable ALS. Furthermore, the relative restriction of lower motor neuron signs and examination findings in the lower extremities should raise the question of a more focal process. On the other hand, over time, this patient may develop more widespread involvement and may develop upper motor neuron signs, such that eventually clinical criteria for probable ALS may be clear-cut.

In patients with a pure lower motor neuron presentation, it is important to consider spinomuscular atrophy, in general a slower form of motor neuron disease associated with abnormalities of the survivor motor neuron gene. Patients with pure lower motor neuron syndromes with bulbar involvement should also be considered for multifocal motor neuropathy. Typically, the patients have marked conduction block on nerve conduction studies, and about half of them demonstrate elevated levels of anti-GM1 antibodies. The diagnosis results in a much more favorable prognosis for patients, and the condition is typically improved with i.v. Ig therapy. Patients with pure lower motor neuron syndrome should be screened for a monoclonal gammopathy with serum protein electrophoresis and related studies, as occasional patients have been observed to stabilize with treatment of an underlying monoclonal disorder.

As with any focal lower motor neuron disturbance, particularly involving paraparesis, meticulous imaging of the spine is mandatory to rule out a structural lesion (a tumor, spinal vascular malformation, syrinx, etc.). Inflammatory disorders of the root, such as an immune-mediated polyradiculopathy or an infectious polyradiculopathy, should be considered and evaluated with spinal fluid studies. An infiltrating process such as sarcoidosis or fungal or carcinomatous meningitis might also affect multiple motor roots and lead to a progressive course, although most patients have symptoms and signs beyond the lower motor neurons.

In this patient, following a thorough laboratory evaluation, the working diagnosis is motor neuron disease. Clearly, such patients require careful long-term monitoring and reevaluation of their clinical status.

Therapy of motor neuron disease is generally divided into two strategies. Strategy one is the treatment of symptoms resulting from the condition; in this patient's case, aggressive rehabilitation measures, including splinting for foot drop and assessment of ambulation and mobility with equipment and safety devices, are a priority. Muscle cramps are treated with quinine. Patients with upper motor neuron disease with substantial spasticity are treated with antispasticity drugs. Patients who develop upper extremity involvement require experienced occupational therapy, including equipment, to facilitate their activities of daily living (ADL) function.

Assessment of forced vital capacity (FVC) looking for diaphragmatic involvement is indicated; when the FVC falls below 60% of predicted, patients should be treated with bilevel positive airway pressure (BIPAP). As patients develop bulbar dysfunction with dysphagia and speech difficulty, symptomatic management with equipment for speech and percutaneous endoscopic gastrostomy (PEG) for dysphagia are indicated. In general, patients are best managed in a multidisciplinary clinic setting in which the various therapies and evaluations can be performed every 3 months.

The second strategy is to treat the underlying motor neuron disturbance. At the present time, the only drug that has been proven in double-blind prospective trials to affect the progression of motor neuron disease is riluzole, which prolongs survival in patients with ALS. There are numerous other investigational agents, but at this time they remain unproven in humans with motor neuron disease.

■ **SELECTED REFERENCES**

Biller J, ed. *Practical neurology,* 2nd ed. Philadelphia: Lippincott Williams & Wilkins, 2002:Chapter 45.
Pascuzzi RM. ALS, motor neuron disease, and related disorders: a personal approach to diagnosis and management. *Semin Neurol* 2002;22:75–87.

■ **SEE QUESTIONS: 1, 5, 11, 15, 18, 77, 173, 186, 214**

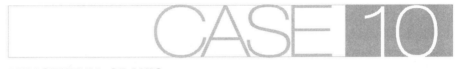

MYASTHENIA GRAVIS

OBJECTIVES

▨ To review the differential diagnosis for fluctuating proximal weakness.
▨ To summarize the diagnostic workup for myasthenia gravis (MG) and Lambert-Eaton syndrome.
▨ To illustrate the evaluation and management of the patient with seronegative myasthenia gravis.
▨ To review treatment options for patients with autoimmune MG.

VIGNETTE

A 43-year-old man, previously healthy, had progressive muscle weakness and fatigability.

CASE SUMMARY

The patient is a 43-year-old man who presents with several months of fluctuating limb weakness, worse with exercise and relatively worse later in the day. The patient has no cranial symptoms. The examination confirms the presence of proximal weakness of the limbs. The history suggests and the examination confirms the presence of fluctuating or fatigable weakness based on response to repetitive exercise.

Although myasthenia gravis presents with fluctuating or fatigable weakness, the majority of patients have significant cranial involvement. Twenty-five percent of patients present with diplopia, 25% with ptosis, and by one month 80% have some degree of ocular involvement. Ten percent of myasthenics present with bulbar symptoms, 10% with lower extremity weakness, and 10% with generalized weakness, whereas respiratory failure is the presenting symptom in 1%.

Lambert-Eaton myasthenic syndrome is far less common than MG and is associated with proximal limb weakness, particularly in the lower extremities, with a relative paucity of cranial weakness. The absence of dry mouth (and other antimuscarinic, anticholinergic symptoms), as well as the preservation of muscle stretch reflexes, would be against Lambert-Eaton myasthenic syndrome in the present patient. An acquired myopathy such as polymyositis, dermatomyositis, inclusion body myositis, or thyroid disease are also in the differential, but far less likely to cause the degree of fluctuation in strength described and shown by this patient. Metabolic or genetic disorders such as adult-onset acid maltase deficiency, follicle-stimulating hormone (FSH) dystrophy, and Desmond myopathy are additional myopathies in the differential.

In this patient serologic studies reveal no detectable acetylcholine receptor antibodies (about 80% sensitive for MG). In addition, there were no detectable anti-PQ type voltage-gated calcium channel antibodies (typically seen in Lambert-Eaton myasthenic syndrome). In patients with suspected autoimmune MG who are seronegative for acetylcholine receptor antibodies, about 50% are estimated to have anti-MuSK antibodies. This patient was seronegative for MuSK antibodies. Pharmacological testing revealed a positive response to cholinesterase inhibitors, supporting a neuromuscular junction diagnosis.

Neurophysiologic studies revealed normal compound muscle action potential (CMAP) amplitudes, normal nerve conduction velocities, and the presence of a decremental response to low rates of repetitive stimulation. The EMG needle examination was normal. The decremental response with normal baseline CMAP amplitudes would favor the presence of myasthenia gravis. In Lambert-Eaton syndrome the baseline motor amplitudes are uniformly low. Therefore the clinical presentation, response to cholinesterase inhibitors, and neurophysiologic studies lead to a diagnosis of myasthenia gravis.

Management of MG includes the use of cholinesterase inhibitors as first-line therapy, performance of a thymectomy in patients with suspected thymoma or those with moderate to severe weakness, and the use of immunosuppressive therapy. The patient's limited response to cholinesterase inhibitors and the severity of weakness with limitation of function led to the performance of a thymectomy with histological findings of thymic hyperplasia. The response to thymectomy tends to be delayed one or more years following the procedure. The patient was therefore treated with immunosuppressive therapy, in this case mycophenolate mofetil, with improvement in strength 1 to 2 months after initiating therapy.

■ **SELECTED REFERENCES**

Pascuzzi RM. Pearls and pitfalls in the diagnosis and management of neuromuscular junction disorders. *Semin Neurol* 2001;21:425–440.
Sanders DB, El-Salem K, Massey JM, et al. Clinical aspects of MuSK antibody positive seronegative MG. *Neurology* 2003;60:1978–1980.

■ **SEE QUESTIONS: 1, 2, 11, 12, 13, 18, 73, 74**

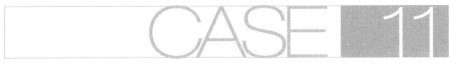

MYOTONIC DYSTROPHY

OBJECTIVES

- To recognize the importance of examining the mother in evaluating a floppy or weak newborn.
- To recognize the classical facies of myotonic dystrophy and illustrate the clinical phenomena of grip myotonia and percussion myotonia.
- To emphasize the systemic complications of myotonic dystrophy.
- To list the differential diagnosis of myotonic dystrophy including current subtypes.

VIGNETTE

A 31-year-old woman gave birth to a hypotonic baby.

CASE SUMMARY

This 31-year-old woman gave birth to a floppy baby 2 weeks ago. Although the mother has no past neurological or neuromuscular history of symptoms, simple observation reveals classic features of myotonic dystrophy with a myopathic lugubrious facies and mild ptosis. In addition, the patient demonstrates a classic grip and percussion myotonia. In men, the diagnosis can be even more obvious given the presence of frontal balding. Ninety percent of patients have cataracts. Myotonic dystrophy typically produces substantial distal weakness, often more pronounced than in proximal muscle groups. Myotonic dystrophy is often referred to as one of the distal myopathies.

The diagnosis is usually obvious from the examination and family history, but mild or atypical cases may require laboratory investigation. Myotonic dystrophy type 1 is associated with an abnormal CTG trinucleotide repeat on chromosome 19. Myotonic dystrophy is associated with EMG changes of myotonic discharges and small myopathic voluntary motor units.

The importance of making a diagnosis is twofold. Myotonic dystrophy patients acquire numerous systemic complications. Cardiac conduction abnormalities can be life threatening (and preventable). Obstructive and central sleep apnea, endocrinopathies, dysphagia, gallbladder disease, and learning disabilities are examples of relatively common associated disorders. The second important aspect of making the diagnosis in this autosomal dominant condition is the fact that many patients are unaware that they have the disease (therefore, examination of relatives is indicated).

The treatment remains symptomatic, including equipment to help with ADLs such as ankle-foot orthosis (AFOs). Screening and management of cardiac disease, respiratory insufficiency, and gastrointestinal involvement should be included in the long-term evaluation and management plan. Myotonia in such patients is usually not so disabling as to require membrane stabilizing medication. As the patients age, their myotonia becomes less pronounced.

The differential diagnosis includes proximal myotonic myopathy (PROMM), which is similar in clinical appearance to myotonic dystrophy except that patients tend not to have distal weakness (instead, weakness is proximal), and PROMM patients tend to have more symptomatic muscle stiffness from myotonia. Myotonic dystrophy type 2 is clinically similar to type 1 other than a tendency to have a mixture of proximal and distal weakness; also, type 2 is associated with a different expansion than that of myotonic dystrophy type 1.

Congenital myotonic dystrophy should be considered in any floppy baby or weak newborn. It is the most severe form of the disease and typically inherited from the mother. The best diagnostic test is a brief evaluation of the infant's mother (as in the presented video). Myotonia congenita is a benign autosomal dominant condition involving more severe muscle stiffness and myotonia but without systemic complications or progressive weakness. Such patients often do require and respond to membrane stabilizing medications such as anticonvulsants. Such patients often have bulky muscles as opposed to atrophy.

■ SELECTED REFERENCES

Biller J, ed. *Practical neurology,* 2nd ed. Philadelphia: Lippincott Williams & Wilkins, 2002:Chapter 47.
Thornton C. The myotonic dystrophies. *Semin Neurol* 1999;19:25–33.

■ SEE QUESTIONS: 1, 58, 77, 202

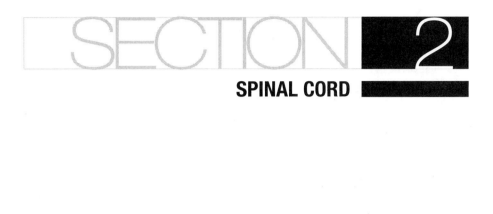

SPINAL CORD

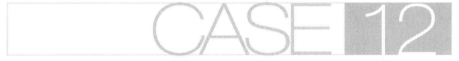

POSTTRAUMATIC CERVICAL SYRINGOMYELIA

OBJECTIVES

▦ To describe a patient with posttraumatic cervical spinal cord dysfunction.
▦ To review the classification of syringomyelia and different conditions associated with this entity.

VIGNETTE

In 1960 this 65-year-old woman became instantly paralyzed from the neck down after a diving accident when she hit the bottom of the pool. Two days later she had an emergency cervical laminectomy. She was then placed on tongs and gradually improved her sensation and movement, more in the arms than in her legs. However, she subsequently developed sequelae of a motor deficit on the right side of her body and a sensation deficit on the left side of her body, particularly to pain and hot and cold temperatures.

CASE SUMMARY

Several years after sustaining a serious high cervical spinal cord injury that initially rendered her quadriplegic, and following a very satisfactory recovery after emergency cervical laminectomy, our patient developed a progressive neurologic syndrome characterized by decreased mobility on the right side of her body, particularly affecting the intrinsic muscles of her right hand. She also had lost the normal feeling of pain, hot, and cold on the left side. She did not complain of brachialgia or shoulder pain.

   Examination was remarkable for contractures, impaired dexterity, and muscular atrophy of her right hand causing a *main en griffe* (clawhand) appearance, right-sided long-tract signs, and loss of pain and temperature appreciation on the left side (not shown on the tape) without a classical cape or hemicape distribution. There was no right-sided segmental anesthesia, facial analgesia, or thermal hypesthesia. She had preservation of light-touch sensation, position sense, and vibration sense. There was no evidence of a Horner syndrome, brainstem findings, scoliosis, digital ulcerations, or Charcot joint deformities.

Our patient had cervical spinal cord dysfunction due to a central cord syndrome associated with a characteristic sensory dissociation syndrome manifested by loss of pain and heat and cold sensations, with sparing of touch, vibration, and position sense (syringomyelic dissociation). In addition to the cervical postlaminectomy changes, MRI showed a tubular cystic cavitation of the spinal cord extending from C-3 through C-7, consistent with the diagnosis of syringohydromyelia, also known as hydrosyringomyelia. There was no Chiari malformation or other extrinsic lesion at the level of the foramen magnum. The syrinx did not communicate with the IV ventricle. There was no evidence of intramedullary mass lesion nor MRI changes suggestive of adhesive spinal arachnoiditis. There was no evidence of basilar impression or platybasia. A final diagnosis of posttraumatic noncommunicating syringohydromyelia was reached.

Syringomyelia may present with confusing unilateral symptoms such as segmental limb hypertrophy rather than segmental amyotrophy, which is a common feature from extension of the syrinx into the anterior horn cells. A neuropathic shoulder arthropathy may be a feature of syringomyelia. Scoliosis in childhood may develop secondary to syringomyelia; syringomyelic deformities tend to be kyphoscoliotic. An isolated Horner syndrome may be a presenting feature. Isolated segmental myoclonus and periodic limb movements have been described. Respiratory failure, postural tachycardia, and gastrointestinal dysfunction may be associated with syringomyelia.

A central cord syndrome is seen in syringomyelia (syringohydromyelia) and trauma. Syringomyelia is a chronic cavitating disorder of the spinal cord, usually located at the lower cervical or upper thoracic spinal cord level, which causes a progressive myelopathy. Syringomyelia has been associated with hindbrain malformations (Chiari I malformation without hydrocephalus and Chiari II malformation with hydrocephalus), spinal cord tumors (particularly intramedullary cervical spinal cord tumors), chronic adhesive spinal arachnoiditis (postoperative, postinfectious, postsubarachnoid hemorrhage), and trauma. Terminal syringomyelia has been associated with the tethered cord syndrome. The term *idiopathic syringomyelia* is applied when no cause is found; idiopathic syringomyelia is very rare.

Classically, syringomyelia has been classified into the following varieties: (i) communicating, (ii) posttraumatic, (iii) tumor related, (iv) arachnoiditis related, and (v) idiopathic. Posttraumatic syringomyelia may develop months to years after a spinal cord injury. Enlarging posttraumatic syringomyelia is manifested clinically by a progressive neurologic deficit that extends some distance above the initial site of injury. When syringomyelia or other intramedullary process is suspected, MRI is the diagnostic procedure of choice. MRI is also useful for the postoperative evaluation of these patients. Treatment of syringomyelia involves a variety of surgical options, depending on the neuroimaging features of the syrinx and its pathogenesis.

■ **SELECTED REFERENCES**

Asano M, Fujiwara K, Yonenobu K, et al. Post-traumatic syringomyelia. *Spine* 1996;21:1446–1453.

Barnett HJM, Foster JB, Hudgson D. *Syringomyelia.* London: WB Saunders, 1973.

Olivero WC. Pathogenesis of syringomyelia. *Am J Neuroradiol* 1999;20:2024–2025.

Schwartz ED, Falcone SF, Quencer RM, et al. Post-traumatic syringomyelia: pathogenesis, imaging, and treatment. *AJR Am J Roentgenol* 1999;173:487–492.

■ **SEE QUESTIONS: 14, 15, 35, 39, 58, 212**

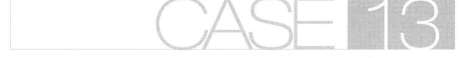

LUMBAR MYELOMENINGOCELE/SPINA BIFIDA

OBJECTIVES

▒ To present an adult patient with sequelae of surgically corrected lumbosacral myelomeningocele.

▒ To review the different entities associated with spinal dysraphism or myelodysplasia.

▒ To emphasize the urologic morbidity associated with myelodysplasia.

VIGNETTE

A 50-year-old woman was evaluated because of gait difficulties.

CASE SUMMARY

Our patient had a history of a lumbosacral myelomeningocele (L5-S1) repaired at the age of 3 months, with subsequent neurogenic bladder and recurrent urinary tract infections and pyelonephritis. She also had a history of syringomyelia and Chiari malformation. The patient currently voided spontaneously with Crede maneuver and catheterized herself intermittently. Several postvoid residuals were in the range of 100 to 200 cc. She also had some degree of rectal incontinence.

There was a history of left club foot repair at the age of 3 years and right fifth toe partial amputation secondary to osteomyelitis. She had required numerous tendon transfers. Her examination demonstrated residual lower extremity paresis, variable loss of sensation in an L5-S1 distribution, and decreased sensation over sacral dermatomes (S3-4 distribution, not shown), and foot deformities. Achilles tendon reflexes were absent bilaterally. MRI showed postoperative changes but no evidence of tethering of the cord.

Our patient has myelodysplasia or spinal dysraphism. This term includes a group of developmental disorders that result from defects in neural tube closure. Closure of the spinal canal begins at the cephalad end on approximately day 20 after fertilization, proceeds caudally, and is complete by approximately day 28. The cause of spinal dysraphism is unknown; genetic and environmental influences have been implicated. Its incidence appears to be increased among the offspring of mothers who had folic acid deficiency during pregnancy.

Most caudal neural tube closure defects occur in the lumbar region. Involvement above L-3, in general, preclude ambulation. Involvement below S-1 allows for un-aided ambulation. Patients with lesions between L-3 and S-1 require assisting devices for ambulation. Patients with myelodysplasia have considerable urologic morbidity. Children with myelodysplasia often have disturbances of bowel function as well.

Lesions of myelodysplasia may include spina bifida occulta, meningocele, myelomeningocele, or lipomyelomeningocele. Spina bifida occulta refers to congen-ital defects of spinal column formation without involvement of the spinal cord or meninges. In many of these patients a cutaneous abnormality (i.e., tuft of hair, cu-taneous angioma or lipoma, or dermal sinus tract) may overlie the lower spine. A meningocele occurs when the meningeal sac extends beyond the confines of the vertebral canal but does not contain neural elements. A myelomeningocele occurs when neural tissue (spinal cord tissue, nerve roots, or both) is included in the sac. A lipomyelomeningocele is defined by the presence of fatty tissue and neural elements within the sac.

Myelomeningoceles account for most of the dysraphic states. The incidence ranges from one case per 1,000 live births in the United States to almost 9 per 1,000 in Ireland. The incidence is lower in Asian countries. Virtually all affected neonates have abnormal bladder function. Most children with a myelomeningocele have an associated Chiari II malformation.

■ SELECTED REFERENCES

Bruner JP, Tulipan N, Paschall RL, et al. Fetal surgery for myelomeningocele and the incidence of shunt-dependent hydrocephalus. *JAMA* 1999;282:1819–1825.

Elwood JH, Nevin NC. Factors associated with anencephalus and spina bifida in Belfast. *Br Prev Med* 1973;27:73–86.

McLone DG. Results of treatment of children born with a myelomeningocele. *Clin Neurosurg* 1983;30:407–412.

Sutherland RS, Mevorach RA, Baskin LS, et al. Spinal dysraphism in children: an overview and an approach to prevent complications. *Urology* 1995;46(Sep):294–304.

■ SEE QUESTIONS: 85, 192, 226, 238

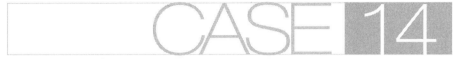

CERVICAL MYELOPATHY (SARCOIDOSIS)

OBJECTIVES

▓ To emphasize the rarity of sarcoidosis exclusively manifested by a myelopathy.
▓ To discuss the differential diagnosis of an expanding intramedullary mass.
▓ To highlight the importance of careful systemic examination in patients with unexplained myelopathy.
▓ To review current treatment for sarcoid myelopathy.

VIGNETTE

A 44-year-old woman had a history of progressive hand numbness and pain. Four years ago she began to experience tingling in the medial aspect of the left hand. The tingling had progressed to involve her entire left hand and the fourth and fifth fingers of her right hand. She also complained of electric shocklike pains down the medial aspect of both arms. She noted that with hot water her symptoms are worse. She had difficulty in writing and holding objects. She can no longer exercise.

The pain comes in waves that last approximately 15 minutes and then eases up. The pain is worse when she is hugged. She has not experienced any visual changes or double vision. She has not experienced any outright weakness, dysarthria, or vertigo. Her bowels and urinary system continue to work well.

CASE SUMMARY

Our patient presented with a subacute cervical myelopathy. A spinal cord tumor was initially suspected by the referring physician. MRI of the spinal cord showed an intramedullary enhancing mass accompanied by expansile surrounding edema from the C-3 to C-7 level. Radiological differential diagnosis included ependymoma, demyelinating disease, multiple sclerosis, metastasis, or transverse myelitis. MRI of the brain showed no intracranial mass, abnormal parenchymal or leptomeningeal enhancement, or other focal abnormalities. The cerebellar tonsils were borderline low. Chest radiograph showed bilateral hilar and right paratracheal lymphadenopathy. Pathological findings of the skin biopsy were consistent with those of sarcoidosis.

Sarcoidosis is a chronic multisystem granulomatous disease characterized by non-caseating granulomatous reaction of unknown origin. It most frequently involves the lymph nodes and lungs, but any organ can be involved. Involvement of the nervous system represents 5% to 15% of cases. Neurological involvement in the form of myelopathy is one of the rarest manifestations of the disease, affecting less than 0.5% of patients with sarcoidosis. Granulomatous inflammation of the spinal cord and meninges may produce isolated mass lesions or multiple patchy lesions and meningitis. Previous or concurrent skin lesions and eye involvement (i.e., iritis, uveitis) should assist with diagnosis.

Past history of unexplained cranial neuropathies, aseptic meningitis, or hypothalamic/pituitary dysfunction should raise suspicion. Differential diagnosis of sarcoidosis includes indolent malignancies such as lymphoma, tuberculosis, fungal infections, and other smoldering granulomatous conditions. Thus, there is no substitute for a tissue diagnosis. Whenever possible, tissue should be obtained in an effort to secure the diagnosis. The importance of searching other locations that are easier and safer to biopsy than the spinal cord itself must be stressed. If there is no readily accessible biopsy site, a blind biopsy of skeletal muscle may be positive in approximately half of the patients.

It has also been suggested that in patients suspected of spinal cord sarcoidosis from MRI findings, a transbronchial lung biopsy be attempted, even if chest roentgenograms or chest CT are normal. Laboratory data supporting the diagnosis of sarcoidosis include elevation of blood and CSF angiotensin-converting enzyme (ACE) levels and the presence of hilar lymphadenopathy on chest imaging. Elevation of CSF globulin or gamma globulin has been reported in cases of progressive myelopathy due to sarcoidosis.

The clinical course is highly variable, including exacerbations and spontaneous remissions. The mainstay of treatment is corticosteroids. In general, patients with spinal cord involvement have an impressive and relative rapid improvement of clinical and radiographic manifestations when treated with corticosteroids.

■ SELECTED REFERENCES

Delaney P. Neurologic manifestations of sarcoidosis. Review of the literature with a report of 23 cases. *Ann Intern Med* 1977;87:336–346.

Morimoto T, Takeuchi K, Morikawa T, et al. Spinal cord sarcoidosis without abnormal shadows on chest radiography or chest CT diagnosed by transbronchial lung biopsy. *Nihon Kokyuki Gakkai Zasshi* 2001;39:871–876.

Pierre-Kahn V, Capelle L, Sbai A, et al. Intramedullary spinal cord sarcoidosis. Case report and review of the literature. *Neurochirurgie* 2001;47:439–441.

Stern BJ, Krumholz A, Johns C, et al. Sarcoidosis and its neurological manifestations. *Arch Neurol* 1985;42:909–917.

■ SEE QUESTIONS: 10, 12, 17, 39, 58, 190, 240

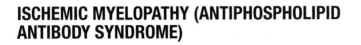

ISCHEMIC MYELOPATHY (ANTIPHOSPHOLIPID ANTIBODY SYNDROME)

OBJECTIVES

▓ To review the arterial blood supply of the spinal cord.
▓ To discuss the main clinical features of spinal cord infarction in the distribution of the anterior spinal artery.
▓ To summarize the main etiologies of arterial spinal cord infarction.
▓ To remind clinicians of unusual coagulopathies as the etiology of arterial spinal cord infarction.

VIGNETTE

A 48-year-old woman was evaluated because of bilateral lower extremity weakness and flexion spasms of both legs. During the daytime, she needs to catheterize herself every 2 hours.

CASE SUMMARY

Our patient had a spinal cord infarction (SCI). Initial investigations were geared to exclude the most common causes of a rapidly producing partial transverse spinal cord lesion, such as cord compression, spinal cord trauma, acute parainfectious or demyelinating myelopathy, and central cord syndromes caused by tumors or hemorrhages. SCI is an uncommon but often devastating disease. Arterial SCI can occur when the blood supply to the spinal cord is interrupted anywhere from the aorta to the intramedullary vasculature by vessel occlusion (thrombotic or embolic), inadequate systemic perfusion pressure, or a combination of both mechanisms.

Three basic vascular systems supply the spinal cord: (i) three spinal arteries (a single anterior spinal artery and paired posterior spinal arteries), (ii) radicular arteries, and (iii) terminal extramedullary and intramedullary arteries. The anterior spinal artery arises from the two intracranial vertebral arteries and descends in the anterior sulcus of the spinal cord, supplying the anterior two-thirds of the spinal cord including the anterior horns, corticospinal tracts, and lateral spinothalamic tracts. The two posterior spinal arteries also most commonly arise from the vertebral arteries and descend along the posterior surface of the spinal cord as an anastomotic network. The posterior spinal arteries supply the posterior one-third of the spinal cord including the dorsal columns.

The anterior and posterior spinal arteries join in an anastomotic loop at the conus medullaris. Only a few radicular arteries supply the spinal cord. Among those, the arteria radicularis magna or artery of Adamkiewicz supplies the lower anterior thoracic and lumbosacral spinal cord. This artery arises from the aorta and generally enters the spinal canal on the left side (T11-L2 in 60% and T8-10 in 40% of people). The extramedullary and intramedullary systems are the terminal branches supplying the spinal cord; they are made up of the peripheral vasocorona that encircles the spinal cord and the central or sulcal arteries arising from the anterior spinal artery.

The spectrum of spinal cord vascular disease is broad. It covers thrombotic and embolic (arterial or venous) infarctions; lacunar infarctions; transient ischemic attacks (TIAs, embolic or hemodynamic); hematomyelia; epidural, subdural, and subarachnoid hemorrhage; and vascular malformations. This syndrome produces paralysis and loss of pain and temperature sensation below the level of the infarction but spares position, vibration, and light touch. Bladder and bowel function are impaired. There may be associated radicular or girdle pain. The diagnosis of SCI should be considered in a patient with acute onset of neurologic motor or sensory deficit below the neck, especially if it is associated with back pain.

In other instances, the onset and evolution of symptoms is more gradual as occurs with hypoxic myelopathy, which presents as slowly evolving paraparesis or quadriparesis, and the entity known as spinal cord claudication, which is triggered by exertion. The anterior spinal artery syndrome most commonly occurs in the watershed areas or boundary zones where the distal branches of the major arterial systems of the spinal cord anastomose, between the T-1 and T-4 segments and at the L-1 segment. The major clinical syndrome of arterial SCI is the anterior spinal artery syndrome.

Aortic disease is the most common cause of spinal cord ischemia. Causes of thrombotic or hemodynamic arterial SCI include the following: atherosclerotic disease of the aorta, profound and sustained arterial hypotension (i.e., cardiac arrest, sepsis), aortic surgery, occlusive disease of the aorta, diabetes, syphilitic arteritis, tuberculous arteritis, vasculitis, carcinomatous meningitis, hypertensive small vessel disease, aortic dissection, subarachnoid hemorrhage, sickle cell anemia, vertebral artery dissection or occlusion, cervical spondylosis, spinal fracture or dislocation, lumbar sympathectomy, Caisson's disease (decompression sickness), esophageal surgery, and antiphospholipid antibody syndrome. Main causes of embolic arterial SCI include the following: aortic emboli, cholesterol emboli, saddle emboli, fibrocartilaginous emboli, atrial myxoma, aortic or spinal cord angiography, and intraaortic balloon counterpulsation.

Magnetic resonance imaging of the spinal cord is considered mandatory and is the procedure of choice to exclude a compressive lesion masquerading as spinal cord ischemia. If it is not available, then simple radiographs followed by spinal CT myelography should be performed. Once spinal cord compression has been ruled out, a lumbar puncture can be performed to exclude inflammatory, infectious, or neoplastic processes.

After extensive evaluation, our patient was found to have persistent elevations of antiphospholipid antibodies titer. Her SCI was attributed to a prothrombotic state due to a primary antiphospholipid antibody syndrome (APAS). Reported neurologic involvement associated with antiphospholipid antibodies includes ischemic strokes, TIAs, ocular ischemia, migrainous-like events, cerebral venous thrombosis, dementia (with or without Sneddon syndrome), acute ischemic encephalopathy, transient global amnesia, seizures, chorea, Guillain-Barré syndrome, and transverse myelopathy. It is generally accepted that oral anticoagulation with warfarin is the preferred treatment for the prevention of thromboembolic events in patients with APAS. Our patient received warfarin.

■ SELECTED REFERENCES

Cuadrado MJ, Hughes GRV. Antiphospholipid (Hughes) syndrome. *Rheum Dis Clin North Am* 2001;27: 507–524.
Lynch DR, Galette SL. Spinal cord ischemia. In: Feldmann E. *Current diagnosis in neurology.* St. Louis, MO: Mosby, 1994:51–57.
Satran R. Spinal cord infarction. *Curr Concepts Cerebrovasc Dis Stroke* 1987;22:13–17.
Williams LS, Bruno A, Biller J. Spinal cord infarction. *Top Stroke Rehabil* 1996;3(Jan):41–53.

■ SEE QUESTIONS: 10, 12, 14, 18

CASE 16

PARAPARESIS AFTER NITROUS OXIDE ANESTHESIA

OBJECTIVES

▓ To emphasize a rare neurological complication of nitrous oxide exposure.
▓ To discuss the differential diagnosis of cobalamin deficiency.
▓ To remind the practitioner that nitrous oxide can cause cobalamin deficiency.
▓ To highlight the importance of careful assessment of vitamin B_{12} levels prior to any exposure to nitrous oxide.

VIGNETTE

A 46-year-old previously healthy man began experiencing abdominal pain and loose stools. He was admitted to the hospital and found to the have an increased white blood count (WBC). He had a sigmoid colon resection with a colostomy. He had epidural anesthesia and also received general anesthesia with nitrous oxide.

Following surgery, he had weakness of both lower extremities, numbness on his feet up to his ankles bilaterally, lack of bladder control, and impaired erections.

CASE SUMMARY

A nonvegan man with a possible subclinical cobalamin (vitamin B_{12}) deficiency developed lower extremity weakness and numbness, loss of bladder control, and impaired erections after exposure to nitrous oxide anesthesia. He also had received epidural anesthesia. Examination demonstrated predominantly distal lower extremity paresis, patellar hyperreflexia, Achilles areflexia, and sensory changes on an L5-S1 distribution. He also had bilateral extensor plantar responses (not shown on the tape). MRI of the thoracic and lumbosacral spine showed a tiny amount of posterior epidural fluid collection at the T12-L1 level, probably representing a resolving discrete epidural hematoma.

EMG findings were consistent with an acute bilateral lumbosacral radiculopathy involving the L5-S1 nerve roots. Urodynamic studies showed a hypotonic noncompliant neurogenic bladder with intact sensation. He was found to have low concentrations of serum vitamin B_{12}. We interpreted his clinical and laboratory findings as strong evidence of a myeloneuropathy due to exposure to nitrous oxide in an individual who had subclinical vitamin B_{12} deficiency. We felt it was quite unlikely that the small epidural hematoma noted on MRI accounted for his myeloneuropathy.

The most common cause of cobalamin deficiency is pernicious anemia due to autoimmune parietal cell dysfunction, associated with defective gastric secretion and absence of intrinsic factor. Cobalamin deficiency may also be caused by inadequate dietary intake (vegans), atrophy of the gastric mucosa, partial or total gastrectomy, functionally abnormal intrinsic factor, inadequate proteolysis of dietary cobalamin, insufficient pancreatic protease, bacterial overgrowth in the intestine, terminal ileum disease, tapeworm infection, disorders of plasma transport of cobalamin, dysfunctional uptake and use of cobalamin by cells, and nitrous oxide administration.

Classic pernicious anemia produces cobalamin deficiency due to failure of the stomach to secrete intrinsic factor. Pernicious anemia is also associated with other autoimmune diseases, such as Addison's disease, Graves' disease, and hypoparathyroidism. In pernicious anemia, the neurological manifestations reflect myelin degeneration of the dorsal and lateral columns of the spinal cord, peripheral nerve dysfunction, and cerebral dysfunction.

Neurological symptoms include paresthesias of toes and fingers, weakness, clumsiness, distal loss of proprioception, and unsteady gait. Loss of position sense in the second toe and loss of vibratory sense for a 256-Hertz but not a 128-Hertz tuning fork are the earliest signs of dorsolateral column involvement. Loss of mental capacities, confusion, irritability, memory impairment, perversion of taste and smell, diminished visual acuity, optic atrophy, and impaired micturition may occur as well.

Nitrous oxide is widely used in anesthesia. Nitrous oxide is a potent oxidant that has multiple deleterious effects on cobalamin metabolism. In humans, the use of nitrous oxide is associated with neurologic and hematologic abnormalities. Patients with unrecognized cobalamin deficiency may be particularly susceptible to brief exposures to nitrous oxide, which inactivates cobalamin-dependent methionine synthase and may cause a myeloneuropathy. In healthy subjects, this side effect on the methionine synthase methylcobalamin complex may be well compensated for by the large vitamin B_{12} stores in the liver and bone marrow. For patients with a preexisting vitamin B_{12} deficiency, even a short course of nitrous oxide anesthesia may deplete the few remaining stores.

Furthermore, the inactivation of methionine synthase by nitrous oxide may be more rapid in patients with low concentrations of vitamin B_{12}. Clinicians should be aware of this condition when confronted with patients with a myeloneuropathy after surgical or dental procedures. The risk may be avoided by promptly administering vitamin B_{12} to patients with suspected or confirmed vitamin B_{12} deficiency before surgery involving nitrous oxide anesthesia. Our patient subsequently received intramuscular injections of vitamin B_{12}, 1000 μg daily for 5 days, and then 1000 μg every month. He also received folate replacement therapy.

■ SELECTED REFERENCES

Flippo TS, Holder ED Jr. Neurologic degeneration associated with nitrous oxide anesthesia in patients with vitamin B12 deficiency. *Arch Surg* 1993;128:1391–1395.

Marie RM, Le Biez E, Busson P, et al. Nitrous oxide anesthesia-associated myelopathy. *Arch Neurol* 2000;57:380–382.

McMorrow AM, Adams RJ, Rubenstein MN. Combined system disease after nitrous oxide anesthesia: a case report. *Neurology* 1995;45:1224–1225.

Rosener M, Dichgans J. Severe combined degeneration of the spinal cord after nitrous oxide anaesthesia in a vegetarian. *J Neurol Neurosurg Psychiatry* 1996;60(Mar):354–356.

■ SEE QUESTIONS: 10, 14, 15, 39, 58, 141, 172, 192, 210, 213

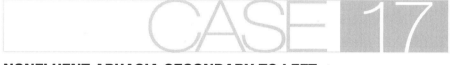

SECTION 3

BEHAVIORAL NEUROLOGY

CASE 17

NONFLUENT APHASIA SECONDARY TO LEFT FRONTAL INFARCTION

OBJECTIVES

- To present characteristic features of Broca's aphasia.
- To name the important components of an examination for aphasias.
- To name the most common types of aphasia.
- To review one of the commonest etiologies of Broca's aphasia.

VIGNETTE

One week after quadruple coronary artery bypass, this 62-year-old man with a history of coronary artery disease, hypertension, hyperlipidemia, and prior left hemispheric cortical infarct developed a sudden onset of language difficulties and right-sided weakness.

CASE SUMMARY

One week following four-vessel coronary artery bypass graft (CABG) surgery, while on 81 mg of aspirin daily, our patient had a sudden onset of language impairment. On arising and going to the restroom, he voided, at which time he had sudden onset of inability to speak. His wife immediately called 911. Past medical history was remarkable for arterial hypertension, hyperlipidemia, three prior myocardial infarctions, and a left parietal ischemic stroke. The patient received intraarterial tissue plasminogen activator (tPA).

On subsequent evaluation, he had nonfluent verbal output. Speech was poorly articulated, effortful, and dysprosodic. He was able to utter the most meaningful words of a sentence, but often omitted the small grammatical words (telegraphic speech or agrammatism). Repetition was impaired. There was a fairly adequate preservation of comprehension of spoken language. He had a faciobrachial distribution of the right hemiparesis. Echocardiography showed left ventricular dilatation, reduced global left ventricular systolic function, left atrial dilatation, regional wall motion abnormality, mild mitral regurgitation, and a thickened aortic valve without significant stenosis. A diagnosis of Broca's aphasia due to a cardioembolic left frontal infarction involving branches of the superior division of the middle cerebral artery (MCA) was made, and warfarin therapy initiated.

Aphasia refers to loss or impairment of language processing caused by brain damage. When assessing language function one must note verbal fluency, auditory comprehension, naming, repetition, reading, and writing. Repetition should include sentences with functor words. "No ifs, ands, or buts" is commonly used. The most common perisylvian aphasias are (i) Broca's aphasia, (ii) Wernicke's aphasia, (iii) global aphasia, and (iv) conduction aphasia. Table 17.1 summarizes the essential features of these aphasias. The other four traditional aphasic syndromes include anomic aphasia and the three types of transcortical aphasias (transcortical motor, transcortical sensory, and mixed transcortical) where repetition is preserved.

Broca's aphasia is characterized by nonfluent verbal output, poor repetition, and relatively intact comprehension of spoken language. Prosody is often disturbed. Writing (even with the nonparalyzed left hand) and oral reading abilities are impaired. Patients with Broca's aphasia are aware of their language deficits and often become frustrated and depressed. Lesions producing this type of aphasia are typically located in the posterior portion of the inferior frontal gyrus, anterior to the motor strip, of the dominant hemisphere. Usually the lesions extend to the neighboring cortex and underlying white matter. The most common cause of Broca's aphasia is arterial occlusion of the left middle cerebral artery branches feeding the posterior portion of the inferior frontal gyrus and the lower portion of the central gyrus.

Wernicke's aphasia is characterized by fluent and effortless speech output, impaired auditory comprehension, and poor repetition. Lesions producing this type of aphasia are typically located in the posterior part of the superior temporal gyrus of the dominant hemisphere. Global aphasia is characterized by nonfluent speech, poor auditory comprehension, and poor repetition. Lesions are typically located throughout the perisylvian region of the dominant hemisphere, encompassing at least part of the frontal, temporal, and parietal lobes. Conduction aphasia is characterized by fairly fluent speech, relatively intact auditory comprehension, but poor repetition.

The arcuate fasciculus connecting Broca's and Wernicke's areas is often involved, but lesions circumscribed to the supramarginal gyrus, primary auditory cortex, and large posterior perisylvian lesions also cause conduction aphasia. In most aphasias, reading impairment and writing impairment parallel oral language comprehension and expression deficits. Paraphasic errors and word-finding difficulties can be seen in many types of aphasia (Table 17.1).

The MCA territory is the most common site of ischemic stroke. The clinical picture of MCA territory infarction varies according to the site of occlusion (e.g., stem, superior division, inferior division, lenticulostriate branches) and the available

TABLE 17.1: NONFLUENT APHASIA SECONDARY TO LEFT FRONTAL INFARCTION

Type	Fluency	Comprehension	Repetition
Broca	**Nonfluent**	**Intact (relative)**	**Impaired**
Wernicke	Fluent	Impaired	Impaired
Global	Nonfluent	Impaired	Impaired
Conduction	Fluent	Intact	Impaired

collaterals. The clinical features of MCA territory infarction are extremely varied [e.g., complete MCA territory, deep territory, superficial anterior (superior) territory, and superficial posterior (inferior) territory]. Embolism of cardiac origin accounts for approximately 15% to 20% of all ischemic strokes. Stroke occurs after CABG with a frequency ranging between 1% and 5%. Two-thirds of strokes occur by the second postoperative day and predominantly involve the cerebral hemispheres.

■ SELECTED REFERENCES

Alexander MP, Benson DF. The aphasias and related disturbances. In: Joynt RJ, ed. *Clinical neurology,* vol 1. Philadelphia: JB Lippincott Co, 1993:1–58.
Biller J, ed. *Practical neurology,* 2nd ed. Philadelphia: Lippincott Williams & Wilkins, 2002:Chapter 3.
Mesulam MM. *Principles of behavioral neurology,* 2nd ed. New York: Oxford, 2000.

■ SEE QUESTIONS: 32, 53, 174

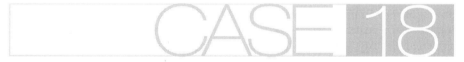

CASE 18

NONFLUENT APHASIA SECONDARY TO LICA OCCLUSION

OBJECTIVES

- ▨ To demonstrate a brief evaluation of a patient with an acute aphasic syndrome.
- ▨ To name the important components of an examination for aphasias.
- ▨ To name the perisylvian aphasias.
- ▨ To analyze the most common characteristics and evolution of global aphasia.

VIGNETTE

A 69-year-old African-American woman with a history of hypertension and diabetes was evaluated because of the sudden onset of speech difficulties.

CASE SUMMARY

Our patient had a sudden onset of language difficulty. She had no preceding TIAs and had a prior history of arterial hypertension and diabetes. The video shown was obtained within 24 hours of symptom onset. On initial evaluation, her spontaneous speech was markedly reduced but not to a state of mutism. She was able to utter only a few words (e.g., well, yes, O.K.). Naming, repetition, and comprehension of spoken language were compromised. Reading and writing (not shown) were also affected. She had a minimal right central facial paresis, a right-hand drift, and a right Babinski sign.

Despite the minimal associated neurologic deficits, her acute aphasia fits best into the category of a nonfluent, nonrepetitive aphasia with impaired comprehension, thus resembling a global aphasia. Further investigations showed an acute left frontal infarction on diffusion-weighted MRI and an occluded cervical left internal carotid artery at its origin.

We suspected intracranial embolism to be the most likely mechanism of her frontal infarction. She was treated with aspirin and received speech therapy. Her aphasia subsequently evolved into the profile of a Broca's aphasia.

Aphasia refers to loss or impairment of language processing caused by brain damage. When assessing language function one must note verbal fluency, auditory comprehension, naming, repetition, reading, and writing. The most common perisylvian aphasias are (i) Broca's aphasia, (ii) Wernicke's aphasia, (iii) global aphasia, and (iv) conduction aphasia.

Table 18.1 summarizes the essential features of these aphasias. The other four traditional aphasic syndromes include anomic aphasia and the three types of transcortical aphasias (transcortical motor, transcortical sensory, and mixed transcortical) where repetition is preserved.

Broca's aphasia is characterized by nonfluent speech, poor repetition, and relatively intact comprehension. Lesions producing this type of aphasia are typically located in the posterior portion of the inferior frontal gyrus of the dominant hemisphere. Wernicke's aphasia is characterized by fluent and effortless speech output, impaired auditory comprehension, and poor repetition. Lesions producing this type of aphasia are typically located in the posterior part of the superior temporal gyrus of the dominant hemisphere. Global aphasia is characterized by nonfluent speech, poor auditory comprehension, and poor repetition. Most patients with classical global aphasia have an associated right hemiplegia, right hemisensory abnormalities, and right homonymous visual field loss (Table 18.1).

Lesions are typically located throughout the perisylvian region of the dominant hemisphere, encompassing at least part of the frontal, temporal, and parietal lobes. Rare cases are reported, however, with global aphasia associated with two discrete lesions in the dominant hemisphere (one frontal and one temporoparietal) but less

TABLE 18.1: NONFLUENT APHASIA SECONDARY TO LICA OCCLUSION

Type	Fluency	Comprehension	Repetition
Broca	Nonfluent	Intact (relative)	Impaired
Wernicke	Fluent	Impaired	Impaired
Global	**Nonfluent**	**Impaired**	**Impaired**
Conduction	Fluent	Intact	Impaired

severe neurologic deficits. The latter situation is usually due to an embolic stroke, but may also occur with intraparenchymal hemorrhages and cerebral metastases. As in the case of our patient, global aphasia may evolve into the profile of a Broca's aphasia. Conduction aphasia is characterized by fairly fluent speech, relatively intact auditory comprehension, but poor repetition.

The arcuate fasciculus connecting Broca's and Wernicke's areas is often involved, but lesions circumscribed to the supramarginal gyrus, primary auditory cortex, and large posterior perisylvian lesions also cause conduction aphasia. In most aphasias, reading impairment and writing impairment parallel oral language comprehension and expression deficits. Paraphasic errors and word-finding difficulties can be seen in many types of aphasia.

Occlusion of the internal carotid artery (ICA) can produce symptoms and signs of infarction in either the middle cerebral artery (MCA), or less commonly, the anterior cerebral artery (ACA) territories, or both. Posterior cerebral artery (PCA) territory infarctions can be seen with ICA occlusion if a fetal origin (from a large posterior communicating artery) of the PCA is present. The sole feature that distinguishes the ICA syndrome from a carotid artery syndrome is the presence of amaurosis fugax. The carotid pulse may be absent ipsilaterally. Horner's syndrome may be present due to oculosympathetic involvement along the carotid artery.

■ SELECTED REFERENCES

Benson DF, Ardila A. *Aphasia: a clinical perspective.* New York: Oxford University Press, 1996.
Biller J, ed. *Practical neurology,* 2nd ed. Philadelphia: Lippincott Williams & Wilkins, 2002:Chapter 3.
Legatt AD, Rubin MJ, Kaplan LR, et al. Global aphasia without hemiparesis: multiple etiologies. *Neurology* 1987;37:201–205.
Mesulam MM. *Principles of behavioral neurology,* 2nd ed. New York: Oxford, 2000.

■ SEE QUESTIONS: 33, 66, 89, 167, 183

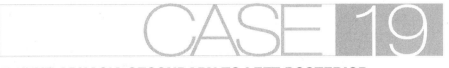

FLUENT APHASIA SECONDARY TO LEFT POSTERIOR TEMPORAL INFARCTION

OBJECTIVES

- To define aphasia.
- To name the important components of an examination for aphasias.
- To name the most common types of aphasia.
- To name the most common anatomic location for each type of aphasia.

VIGNETTE

A 49-year-old right-handed woman, a high school math teacher, without known vascular risk factors, had a sudden onset of speech difficulties and headaches.

CASE SUMMARY

Our patient had a master's degree in math education. She had no prior history of heart disease, arterial hypertension, diabetes, or dyslipidemia. While skiing, she suddenly became disoriented and had trouble remembering her daughter's friend's name. A headache accompanied this. She was taken to the hospital where she was diagnosed with an ischemic stroke. MRI showed ischemic changes in the left posterior temporal region, thought to be embolic in origin, but she had a history of two previous miscarriages, suggesting the possibility of a prothrombotic state.

The patient now complained of residual confusion when writing, spelling, and hunting for words. This was particularly the case with multisyllabic words. She also made mistakes while reading aloud and had difficulty following conversations. She suspected that her memory was reasonably clear for recent details, events, and conversations. She doubted having new problems with mathematics, but she did have trouble remembering phone numbers and quickly transcribing them. She was very much concerned about her ability to return to work, given the state of her language deficits.

On initial evaluation, our patient's conversational speech was unremarkable for dysarthria and prosody was normal. Phrase length was long and language was grammatic, but there were occasional phonemic paraphasias. Letter fluency was impaired. Confrontation naming on the Boston naming test was quite impaired with only 32/60 items named spontaneously and without errors. This improved to 47/60 after self-correction and successive approximation. Comprehension of conversational speech was quite good, but comprehension of syntactically complex or subtly worded questions was clearly impaired.

Writing was marked by good letter formation, although spelling was clearly defective for her level of education. Mental arithmetic was average for age and clearly complicated by poor comprehension, and questions had to be restated several times. Written arithmetic was very well preserved and superior for age. Constructional praxis in assembling blocks to match a template and in copying geometric figures from memory was quite good.

Her aphasia fits best into the category of a fluent aphasia. Further investigations showed hyperhomocysteinemia and transient elevation of β_2 glycoprotein 1 antibodies. She received treatment with aspirin plus clopidogrel and also a combination of folic acid, pyridoxine (vitamin B_6), and cobalamin (vitamin B_{12}).

Aphasia refers to loss or impairment of language processing caused by brain damage. When assessing language function one must note verbal fluency, auditory comprehension, naming, repetition, reading, and writing. Repetition should include sentences with functor words. "No ifs, ands, or buts" is commonly used. The most common aphasias are (i) Broca's aphasia, (ii) Wernicke's aphasia, (iii) global aphasia, and (iv) conduction aphasia. Table 19.1 summarizes the essential features of these aphasias. The other four traditional aphasic syndromes include anomic aphasia and the three types of transcortical aphasias (transcortical motor, transcortical sensory, and mixed transcortical) where repetition is preserved.

Broca's aphasia is characterized by nonfluent speech, poor repetition, and relatively intact comprehension. Lesions producing this type of aphasia are typically located in the posterior portion of the inferior frontal gyrus of the dominant hemisphere. Wernicke's aphasia is characterized by fluent and effortless speech output, impaired auditory comprehension, and poor repetition. Lesions producing this type of aphasia are typically located in the posterior part of the superior temporal gyrus of the dominant hemisphere. Global aphasia is characterized by nonfluent speech, poor auditory comprehension, and poor repetition. Lesions are typically located throughout the perisylvian region of the dominant hemisphere, encompassing at least part of the frontal, temporal, and parietal lobes.

Conduction aphasia is characterized by fairly fluent speech, relatively intact auditory comprehension, but poor repetition. The arcuate fasciculus connecting Broca's and Wernicke's areas is often involved, but lesions circumscribed to the supramarginal gyrus, primary auditory cortex, and large posterior perisylvian lesions also cause conduction aphasia. In most aphasias, reading impairment and writing impairment

TABLE 19.1: FLUENT APHASIA SECONDARY TO LEFT POSTERIOR TEMPORAL INFARCTION

Type	Fluency	Comprehension	Repetition
Broca	Nonfluent	Intact (relative)	Impaired
Wernicke	Fluent	Impaired	Impaired
Global	Nonfluent	Impaired	Impaired
Conduction	**Fluent**	**Intact**	**Impaired**

parallel oral language comprehension and expression deficits. Paraphasic errors and word-finding difficulties can be seen in many types of aphasia.

Commonly used formal scored tests for evaluation of patients with aphasia include the Boston Diagnostic Aphasia Examination (BDAE), the Western Aphasia Battery (WAB), and the Token Test.

■ SELECTED REFERENCES

Biller J, ed. *Practical neurology* 2nd ed. Philadelphia: Lippincott Williams & Wilkins, 2002:Chapter 3.
Mesulam MM. *Principles of behavioral neurology,* 2nd ed. New York: Oxford, 2000.

■ SEE QUESTIONS: 48, 174

CASE 20

WERNICKE APHASIA SECONDARY TO LEFT MCA INFARCTION

OBJECTIVES

- To name the important components of an examination for aphasia.
- To name the most common types of aphasia.
- To name the most common anatomic location for each type of aphasia.
- To present characteristic language abnormalities in a patient with Wernicke's aphasia.

VIGNETTE

A 63-year-old right-handed man, retired construction worker, and part-time professional musician with a history of hypertension and hyperlipidemia presented to his local hospital with a sudden onset of right-sided weakness and language difficulties. He was treated with intravenous tPA.

CASE SUMMARY

Our patient was a retired construction worker and part-time professional musician. He had a history of hypertension and hyperlipidemia. He had a sudden onset of right-sided weakness and language difficulties. At the time of admission to his local emergency room, his blood pressure was 230/120 mm Hg. He received intravenous labetalol, and after a CT scan was obtained, intravenous tPA was administered. The right-sided hemiparesis improved, but his language impairment persisted.

Additional ancillary investigations showed an elevated antinuclear antibody (ANA) (1:2,560) nucleolar pattern and elevated cholesterol, low density lipoprotein (LDL), and triglycerides. Echocardiography showed left ventricular hypertrophy and aortic valve sclerosis, but no evidence of intracardiac thrombi or right-to-left shunt. Carotid ultrasound showed mild plaque formation of both carotid bulbs. MRI showed a large middle cerebral artery territory infarction. MRA showed decreased visualization of a few branches of the left inferior division of the middle cerebral artery. He received antiplatelet therapy, antihypertensives, and a statin. He was referred for further evaluation.

On examination, he was at times anxious and agitated. Verbal output was fluent and phrase lengths of up to 23 words observed. Utterances frequently contained neologistic paraphasias. He also had a number of phonemic paraphasias. Naming and repetition were severely impaired. He could not reliably follow any more than one step command. Comprehension of sentences spoken by others was quite impaired. Comprehension of syntactically complex questions and stories was also quite clearly defective. Reading out loud as well as reading comprehension were abnormal. He could not read simple sentences without being quite paraphasic.

Written expression was accurate for his name but no other autobiographical information. He could not recite automatic sequences (days of the week, months of the year). He could complete simple sentences by selecting the appropriate word, but this quickly became inaccurate with increasing complexity. He attempted to augment the spoken word with spontaneous physical gesture on a number of occasions. He also frequently provided circumlocution/verbal description that was helpful in communicating his message. He also had ideomotor limb apraxia and a residual right superior homonymous quadrantanopia.

In summary, our patient's language impairment was characterized by increased verbal output, impaired repetition, and impaired comprehension of spoken language, characteristic of Wernicke's aphasia. He also had frequent semantic and neologistic paraphasias. A literal paraphasia is when a syllable is substituted within a word (phonemic substitution). Words can be substituted only by meaningless words (neologisms). Further ancillary investigations showed persistent elevations of IgG anticardiolipin (aCL) and antiphosphatidylethanolamine (aPE) antibodies. Antiplatelet therapy was discontinued. He was started on warfarin and referred for speech therapy.

Aphasia refers to loss or impairment of language processing caused by brain damage. When assessing language function one must note verbal fluency, auditory comprehension, naming, repetition, reading, and writing. The most common perisylvian aphasias are (i) Broca's aphasia, (ii) Wernicke's aphasia, (iii) global aphasia, and (iv) conduction aphasia. Table 20.1 summarizes the essential features of these aphasias. The other four traditional aphasic syndromes include anomic aphasia and the three types of transcortical aphasias (transcortical motor, transcortical sensory, and mixed transcortical) where repetition is preserved.

Broca's aphasia is characterized by nonfluent speech, poor repetition, and relatively intact comprehension. Lesions producing this type of aphasia are typically

TABLE 20.1: WERNICKE APHASIA SECONDARY TO LEFT MCA INFARCTION

Type	Fluency	Comprehension	Repetition
Broca	Nonfluent	Intact (relative)	Impaired
Wernicke	**Fluent**	**Impaired**	**Impaired**
Global	Nonfluent	Impaired	Impaired
Conduction	Fluent	Intact	Impaired

located in the posterior portion of the inferior frontal gyrus of the dominant hemisphere. Wernicke's aphasia is characterized by fluent and effortless speech output, impaired auditory comprehension, and poor repetition. The content of speech is often unintelligible because of frequent errors in phonemes and word choices. Lesions producing this type of aphasia are typically located in the posterior part of the superior temporal gyrus of the dominant hemisphere. Wernicke's aphasia most commonly occurs due to infarction in the distribution of the inferior division of the left middle cerebral artery.

Patients with Wernicke's aphasia are often misdiagnosed as having a psychiatric disorder, especially as associated hemiparesis and sensory loss may be absent. Recovery in Wernicke's aphasia is less favorable than in Broca's aphasia. Patients recovering from Wernicke's aphasia may develop the profile of a conduction or anomic aphasia. Global aphasia is characterized by nonfluent speech, poor auditory comprehension, and poor repetition. Lesions are typically located throughout the perisylvian region of the dominant hemisphere, encompassing at least part of the frontal, temporal, and parietal lobes. Conduction aphasia is characterized by fairly fluent speech, relatively intact auditory comprehension, but poor repetition.

The arcuate fasciculus connecting Broca's and Wernicke's areas is often involved, but lesions circumscribed to the supramarginal gyrus, primary auditory cortex, and large posterior perisylvian lesions also cause conduction aphasia. In most aphasias, reading impairment and writing impairment parallel oral language comprehension and expression deficits. Paraphasic errors and word-finding difficulties can be seen in many types of aphasia.

■ SELECTED REFERENCES

Biller J, ed. *Practical neurology,* 2nd ed. Philadelphia: Lippincott Williams & Wilkins, 2002.

Brazis PW, Masdeu JC, Biller J. *Localization in clinical neurology,* 4th ed. Philadelphia: Lippincott Williams & Wilkins, 2001.

Devinsky O. *Behavioral neurology. 100 maxims in Neurology Series,* vol 1. Edward Arnold, 1992:88–90.

Mesulam MM. *Principles of behavioral neurology,* 2nd ed. New York: Oxford, 2000.

■ SEE QUESTIONS: 70, 88, 174, 233

CASE 21

PRIMARY PROGRESSIVE APHASIA

OBJECTIVES

- To present characteristic features of primary progressive aphasia (PPA).
- To analyze the progressive deterioration of PPA.
- To name the most common neuropathologic conditions associated with PPA.

VIGNETTE

Nine years ago, this 72-year-old right-handed man consulted us because of difficulty "coming up with words." Since then, he has had progressive difficulty with several cognitive functions, most specifically forgetting names and nouns and having difficulty reading. His most specific complaint consists of an inability to come up with a specific word even thought he can describe what it means. He has also noticed that he has been forgetting the names of some relatives and friends.

CASE SUMMARY

Our patient was a Ph.D. research physiologist whom we have followed since 1997. Evaluation at that time indicated an anomic aphasia with normal comprehension, anterograde memory, executive function, and visual perception.

Three years later (2000), he described a worsening ability to read and find words and to comprehend certain nouns. His wife also suspected changes in recent memory. Judgment had also apparently changed as he engaged in risky ventures, such as cutting down a tree that his wife warned would land on power lines, which it eventually did. Examination at that time showed well-preserved social graces. Verbal output was largely fluent but showed worsened word-finding difficulties particularly with nouns. Speech was more empty, anomic, and circumlocutory. Occasional semantic paraphasias were also present in conversational speech.

He was able to solve complex and abstract problems nonverbally. There was also mild decline in anterograde visual memory. Constructional praxis remained above average for age but mildly worse than on previous examinations.

One year later (2001), he described himself as feeling quite good, with occasional unhappiness and frustration. He continued to do and enjoy woodworking and mowing the lawn. He nevertheless fell from a ladder when inappropriately standing on the top step and injured his shoulder. His son described this as one of many instances of apparent lack of judgment. Another included filling a lawn mower with a lit cigar in his mouth. Examination revealed an alert and awake man whose affect and mood appeared to be euthymic and reactive. Conversational speech was clearly empty and anomic, with a number of literal and semantic paraphasias. Confrontation naming remained profoundly impaired.

Both reading and written comprehension were clearly disturbed, although reading comprehension was significantly worse. Nonverbal problem solving remained quite good on the Wisconsin Card Sorting test. Nonverbal reasoning with matrices also continued to be quite well preserved. Visual memory for geometric designs was impaired and worse than in previous evaluations.

Our patient experienced onset of a slowly progressive language disorder. He maintained normal cognitive abilities early on in the course of his disease process. Based on the distinctive clinical manifestations, neuropsychological findings, and neuroimaging investigations, we concluded that he had primary progressive aphasia (PPA).

PPA is a distinctive but unusual clinical syndrome characterized by a slow deterioration of language functions with relative preservation of other cognitive functions for at least the first 2 years of the disease process. The disease starts with word-finding disturbances (anomia). Verbal output can be fluent or nonfluent. Personality remains well preserved until advanced stages of the disease. The underlying pathology of PPA is rather heterogeneous. PPA has been linked to variants of frontotemporal degeneration (Pick complex), Alzheimer disease type changes, focal glial tauopathy, corticobasal ganglionic degeneration, progressive supranuclear palsy, focal neuronal achromasia, or lobar atrophy without a distinctive histopathology. Imaging with CT, MRI, single photon emission computed tomography (SPECT), and PET are useful adjuncts for the diagnosis. Differential diagnosis should include slowly progressive aphasias associated with other forms of degenerative brain disorders.

■ SELECTED REFERENCES

Kertesz A, Munoz DG. Primary progressive aphasia. *Clin Neurosci* 1997;4 (2):95–102.

Mesulam MM. Primary progressive aphasia. *Ann Neurol* 2001;49:421–423.

Mesulam MM. *Principles of behavioral neurology,* 2nd ed. New York: Oxford, 2000.

Sobrido MJ, Abu-Khalil A, Weintraub S, et al. Possible association of the tau H1/H1 genotype with primary progressive aphasia. *Neurology* 2003;60:862–864.

■ SEE QUESTIONS: 86, 174

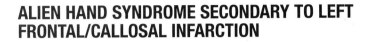

ALIEN HAND SYNDROME SECONDARY TO LEFT FRONTAL/CALLOSAL INFARCTION

OBJECTIVES

▪ To name the three variants of alien hand syndrome.
▪ To recognize the characteristics of the two types of motor alien hand syndrome.

VIGNETTE

A 67-year-old right-handed woman had a 2-year history of progressive abnormal grip and uncontrollable fisting of the right hand.

CASE SUMMARY

The most common lesions originating in the corpus callosum are glioma, lymphoma, and demyelinating disease. Our patient had a striking syndrome secondary to an infarction of the midportion of the corpus callosum and medial aspect of the left frontal lobe, regions supplied by the anterior cerebral artery (ACA). Infarction of the corpus callosum may be more common than previously thought and is often the result of cerebral embolism. Cardioembolism from atrial fibrillation was considered to be the cause of our patient's stroke.

Alien hand syndrome is rare. The term alien hand syndrome was initially used to describe inter-hemispheric disconnection phenomena in patients with lesions of the anterior corpus callosum. Three varieties of alien hand syndrome have been reported: lesions involving the corpus callosum plus dominant medial frontal cortex, lesions involving the corpus callosum alone, and lesions involving posterior cortical and subcortical areas.

Based on the MRI findings and a history of grasping behavior (despite lacking a crural paresis), our patient's intriguing syndrome best fulfills the criteria for a *frontal alien hand syndrome*. This syndrome results from damage to the supplementary motor area, anterior cingulate gyrus, medial prefrontal cortex of the dominant hemisphere, and anterior corpus callosum. The symptoms of the frontal alien hand syndrome always occur in the dominant hand with prominent motor phenomena including reflexive grasping, groping, and compulsive manipulation of tools.

The second type of alien hand syndrome or *callosal alien hand syndrome*, requires only a callosal lesion and is characterized by intermanual conflict with little evidence of limb paresis. Usually the nondominant hand is affected.

The third or *posterior-variant alien hand syndrome* is less frequent and generally involves the nondominant hand, which tends to levitate into the air displaying nonconflictual movements. There is also relevant sensory impairment with triple (sensory, optic, and cerebellar) ataxia and hemispatial neglect.

Alien hand syndrome is usually associated with acute focal lesions such as stroke or surgery of the corpus callosum, but it has also been reported in association with corticobasal ganglionic degeneration, Alzheimer disease, Marchiafava-Bignami disease, Creutzfeldt-Jakob disease, and other chronic dementing diseases, as well as seizures.

■ SELECTED REFERENCES

Giroud M, Dumas R. Clinical and topographical range of callosal infarction: a clinical and radiological correlation study. *J Neurol Neurosurg Psych* 1995;59:238–242.

Marey-Lopez J, Rubio-Nazabal E, Alonso-Magdalena L, et al. Posterior alien hand syndrome after a right thalamic infarct. *J Neurol Neurosurg Psych* 2002;73:447–449.

Suwanwela NC, Lelacheavasit N. Isolated corpus callosal infarction secondary to pericallosal artery disease presenting as alien hand syndrome. *J Neurol Neurosurg Psych* 2002;72:533–536.

■ SEE QUESTION: 253

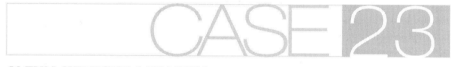

ALEXIA WITHOUT AGRAPHIA

OBJECTIVES

▨ To review the different types of alexias.
▨ To demonstrate an example of alexia without agraphia.

VIGNETTE

A 49-year-old man with a history of poorly controlled hypertension and tobacco abuse presented to the emergency room (ER) 48 hours after the acute onset of chest pain. The patient was taken to the Cardiac Cath lab where he was found to have a right coronary occlusion and left ventricle (LV) thrombus. Immediately following the catheterization, the patient complained of not being able to see. The patient had an emergent cerebral angiogram and received intraarterial tPA followed by integrilin.

This examination is conducted 10 days after the event.

CASE SUMMARY

Our patient had alexia without agraphia and a right homonymous hemianopia. Unless reading and writing are tested, acquired disorders of reading (alexias) and writing (agraphias) are missed. Three types of alexia are recognized: (i) alexia without agraphia, (ii) alexia with agraphia, and (iii) aphasic alexia (frontal or third alexia). Other rare types of alexia include hemialexias following posterior corpus callosum section and unilateral paralexias associated with unilateral inattention syndromes.

As in our patient, infarcts in the distribution of the callosal branches of the PCA involving the left occipital region and the splenium of the corpus callosum produce alexia without agraphia. Alexia without agraphia, first described by Dejerine in 1892, is an isolated inability to read. In this rather striking syndrome, patients can write correctly, speak, and spell normally, but are unable to read words and sentences including their own. The ability to name letters and numbers may be intact, but there can be inability to name colors, objects, and photographs. Alexia without agraphia has been reported with infarcts of the left lingual gyrus with or without involvement of the splenium of the corpus callosum. Dejerine postulated a disconnection syndrome between the intact right visual cortex and the left hemisphere language areas, particularly the angular gyrus.

■ SELECTED REFERENCES

Alexander MP, Benson DF. The aphasias and related disturbances. In: Joynt RJ, ed. *Clinical neurology*, vol 1. Philadelphia: JB Lippincott, 1993:1–58.

Friedman R, Ween JE, Martin AL. Alexia. In: Heilman KM, Valenstein E, eds. *Clinical neuropsychology*. New York: Oxford University Press, 1993.

Geschwind SH. Disconnection syndromes in animals and man. *Brain* 1965;88:237–294, 585–644.

■ SEE QUESTIONS: 34, 52, 53

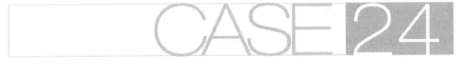

GERSTMANN PLUS SYNDROME

OBJECTIVES

■ To illustrate a reversible angiopathic syndrome of the postpartum period.
■ To review causes of arterial ischemic strokes associated with pregnancy and puerperium.

VIGNETTE

This 38-year-old woman developed headaches in the context of increased blood pressure, approximately 3 days postpartum. She then noticed some visual problems and had spells consisting of word-finding difficulties and right-sided weakness.

CASE SUMMARY

The patient was a 38-year-old left-handed woman (gravida 1, para 0) who, following delivery of healthy twins, developed new onset headaches in the context of increased blood pressure, approximately 3 days postpartum. She had no seizures and had no prior history of migraine headaches.

She was initially diagnosed with migraine headaches and released. No vasoconstrictor drugs had been used, and no medications were given to suppress lactation. She was soon readmitted to the outside hospital with similar complaints and was diagnosed with postpartum preeclampsia. A lumbar puncture showed 19 WBCs, 30 RBCs, a protein of 73, and normal glucose. She was then diagnosed with aseptic meningitis and discharged home.

A few days later, she noticed loss of peripheral vision, spells of word-finding difficulties, and inability to move her right arm. At the time of that admission, she was also reported to have fluctuating blood pressures and a combination of right–left disorientation, finger agnosia, and dyscalculia (Gerstmann described the association of right–left disorientation, finger agnosia, agraphia, and acalculia as characteristic of lesions of the angular and supramarginal gyrus). MRI showed edema in the left posterior head region. MRA revealed multisegmental arterial narrowing of both middle cerebral arteries, both anterior cerebral arteries, and the basilar artery. She was suspected of having an isolated central nervous system (CNS) angiitis and was transferred to our institution for further evaluation.

A repeat lumbar puncture was normal. Transthoracic and transesophageal echocardiographic studies were normal. Extensive investigations for underlying hypercoagulability were unremarkable. Follow up MRI/MRA showed interval evolution of the left posterior parietal-occipital arterial infarct and near complete resolution of vascular irregularities seen on the prior examination. She was diagnosed with probable postpartum cerebral angiopathy. Differential diagnoses included postpartum isolated CNS angiitis and Call-Fleming (reversible sequential cerebral vasoconstriction) syndrome.

The video, obtained a few months after her hospital admission, demonstrated residual neurologic deficits characterized by right–left disorientation, a right inferior homonymous quadrantanopia, and some difficulty with simple arithmetic calculations. She also had right-sided hyperreflexia and a right Babinski sign. She had no obvious naming difficulties, agraphia, or finger agnosia. Her blood pressure had normalized.

Stroke in pregnancy and puerperium encompasses a vast number of clinical phenomena with a diverse array of etiologies (not mutually exclusive). They include the following: thromboembolism, cardioembolism, primary or secondary hypercoagulable states, numerous nonatherosclerotic arteriopathies, arterial hypotension, and various other miscellaneous disorders including preeclampsia/eclampsia, amniotic fluid embolism, migrainous infarction, and cervicocephalic arterial dissections.

There is consensus among recent studies that the immediate postpartum period is a time of higher risk of stroke. A number of studies of stroke in pregnancy have found an association between preeclampsia and eclampsia and stroke. In a recent large case series, hypertensive disorders of pregnancy (including preeclampsia, eclampsia, and the syndrome of hemolysis, elevated liver enzymes, and low platelets known as HELLP syndrome) were a comorbid condition in almost half of the patients with ischemic stroke and in two-thirds of the patients with hemorrhagic stroke.

Cerebral angiopathy in the postpartum period is unusual. The diagnosis is based on clinical findings and angiography. Postpartum cerebral angiopathy (a form of reversible cerebral vasoconstriction) is a poorly defined, reversible clinicoradiologic syndrome characterized by headache, vomiting, seizures, and occasional focal neurologic deficits occurring in the puerperium. A vasoconstrictive response to acute severe hypertension is likely to play a major pathogenetic role in this condition. The neurologic deficits are at times the result of infarction, which tends to predominate in the posterior aspect of the cerebral hemispheres. Some patients have had a history of exposure to ergot derivatives or sympathomimetic agents including bromocriptine, ergonovine, ergometrine maleate, or methylergonovine.

Angiography reveals multisegmental arterial narrowing. As MRA provides excellent imaging of the intracerebral circulation noninvasively, catheter angiography is currently seldom utilized. Transcranial Doppler ultrasound examination is of established value in detecting changes in mean flow velocity and together with MRA allows for noninvasive evaluation of patients with postpartum cerebral angiopathy. Postpartum cerebral angiopathy as a cause of hemorrhagic stroke is unusual. Treatment includes withdrawal of vasoactive substances. The clinical outcome is usually favorable.

Two years later, our patient delivered a healthy baby girl by cesarean section that was induced at the 36th week of gestation. Patients in the general population who suffer a stroke in pregnancy without a specific, identifiable, persistent risk factor for stroke may be at relatively low risk of recurrent stroke in a subsequent pregnancy. When a patient with a history of stroke decides to pursue a pregnancy, pregnancy care should be undertaken in cooperation with a team of physicians including a neurologist and high-risk obstetrician as well as cardiologists, hematologists, and internists, if warranted.

■ SELECTED REFERENCES

Bogousslavsky J, Despland PA, Regli F, et al. Postpartum cerebral angiopathy: reversible vasoconstriction assessed by transcranial Doppler ultrasounds. *Eur Neurol* 1989;29:102–105.

David EF, Wityk RJ. Cerebrovascular disorders. In: *Cherry and Merkatz's complications of pregnancy.* Philadelphia: Lippincott Williams & Wilkins, 2000:465–485.

Donaldson JO. Eclampsia and postpartum cerebral angiopathy. *J Neurol Sci* 2000;178(Sep):1.

Kittner SJ, Stern BJ, Feeser BR, et al. Pregnancy and the risk of stroke. *N Engl J Med* 1996;335:768–774.

■ SEE QUESTIONS: 20, 34, 52, 94

CASE 25

ANTERIOR OPERCULAR SYNDROME (FOIX-CHAVANY-MARIE)

OBJECTIVES

▨ To review the clinical characteristics of a vasculopathic anterior opercular (Foix-Chavany-Marie) syndrome.
▨ To describe nonvascular etiologies of the anterior opercular (Foix-Chavany-Marie) syndrome.

VIGNETTE

A 53-year-old man with a history of diabetes, hypertension, cigarette smoking and remote right MCA infarct with residual left hemiparesis had a sudden onset of slurred speech and right-sided weakness. Due to difficulties handling secretions, he had a tracheostomy and PEG placement at the local hospitals. Due to clinical deterioration, he was transferred for further evaluation.

CASE SUMMARY

Our patient had multiple vascular risk factors including diabetes mellitus, arterial hypertension, and cigarette smoking. He had a previous right middle cerebral artery (MCA) distribution infarct with a residual left hemiparesis. He then experienced acute onset of right-sided weakness and slurred speech. On admission to the local hospital, he was noted to be severely dysarthric with a decreased gag reflex and severely impaired swallowing. As he became unable to handle his own secretions, he had a tracheostomy and placement of a PEG tube. He was then transferred for further evaluation and management.

Subsequent examination was remarkable for adequate verbal comprehension, a positive snout reflex, bilateral palmomental reflexes, bilateral central facial weakness with preservation of emotional facial movements, and bilateral hemiparesis (right hemibody involved to a greater extent than the left hemibody). He was unable to open his mouth or protrude or move his tongue on command. On repeated occasions, he was observed to yawn spontaneously. Due to his tracheostomy, we were unable to assess whether he was anarthric or severely dysarthric. Diffusion-weighted MRI showed signal changes consistent with an acute left anterior opercular infarct and an old right opercular infarct. MRA showed an occluded left internal carotid artery.

The anterior opercular syndrome (Foix-Chavany-Marie syndrome or the syndrome of faciopharyngoglossomasticatory diplegia with automatic voluntary movement dissociation) is a corticosubcortical type of suprabulbar palsy due to bilateral anterior perisylvian lesions involving the primary cortex and parietal opercula. Patients with this syndrome lose voluntary control of facial, pharyngeal, lingual, masticatory, and sometimes ocular muscles. Reflexive and automatic functions of these muscles are preserved. These patients may blink, laugh, or yawn spontaneously, but they cannot open their mouth or close their eyes on command. They do not have emotional lability. The gag reflex is decreased and swallowing is severely impaired. Patients with the anterior opercular syndrome may be distinguished from patients with Broca's aphasia, oral-buccal apraxia, pseudobulbar palsy, or bulbar palsy.

The Foix-Chavany-Marie syndrome has been most often described in association with bilateral vascular lesions of the opercula or their corticofugal projections. Besides vascular etiologies, the anterior opercular syndrome has also been associated with developmental bilateral perisylvian cortical polymicrogyria or central macrogyria, meningoencephalitis, herpes simplex encephalitis, trauma, and neurodegenerative disorders. A reversible form has also been reported in children with epilepsy.

■ SELECTED REFERENCES

Brazis PW, Masdeu JC, Biller J. *Localization in clinical neurology,* 4th ed. Philadelphia: Lippincott Williams & Wilkins, 2001.

Graff-Radford NR, Bosch EP, Stears JC, et al. Developmental Foix-Chavany-Marie syndrome in identical twins. *Ann Neurol* 1986;20:632–635.

Weller M. Anterior opercular cortex lesions cause dissociated lower cranial nerve palsies and anarthria but no aphasia: Foix-Chavany-Marie syndrome and "automatic voluntary dissociation" revisited. *J Neurol* 1993;240:199–208.

■ SEE QUESTIONS: 33, 49, 66, 115, 116, 117, 118, 120, 122, 123

CASE 26

AMNESIA (PCA INFARCT)

OBJECTIVES

■ To review the anatomic circuits and connecting pathways involved in amnesia.
■ To identify disorders associated with acute onset memory loss.
■ To evaluate the leading causes of amnestic syndromes.

VIGNETTE

A 50-year-old right-handed man had a sudden onset of difficulty in comprehending written words (reading the newspaper), troubles remembering, as well as difficulty naming family members and associates. In addition, he had right-sided headaches and a right visual field impairment. Past medical history was remarkable for hypertension and thrombocytopenia of unknown cause diagnosed in 1970.

CASE SUMMARY

Our patient presented with acute onset of memory loss, anomia, alexia, and a right superior homonymous quadrantanopia consistent with an infarct in the distribution of the left posterior cerebral artery. T2-weighted MRI of the brain showed hyperintensities in the inferomedial left posterior cerebral artery. A follow-up MRI of the brain showed hyperintensities on T2-weighted and fluid-attenuated inversion recovery (FLAIR) images in the left hippocampus, amygdala, and occipital lobe. On diffusion-weighted images these areas showed an increased signal. MRA showed a focal stenosis of the left posterior cerebral artery at the P1-P2 junction.

The patient was initially diagnosed as having herpes simplex encephalitis. Herpes simplex encephalitis, the most common cause of sporadic viral encephalitis, presents with a subacute progressive course of headache, fever, an altered sensorium, seizures, and occasionally focal neurologic deficits (i.e., aphasia). Our patient had no recorded fever. The course of his illness was acute and nonprogressive; he awoke with his deficits. Although herpes viruses have a predilection for the limbic system, involving one or both mesial temporal lobes, involvement of the diencephalons and occipital cortex is rare.

Strokes may cause a number of behavioral changes including amnesia. The posterior cerebral arteries and their branches supply the mammillary bodies, the thalami, and the medial and basal temporal lobes including the hippocampi. Infarcts in the anterior distribution of the left posterior cerebral artery cause verbal and visual amnesia, color anomia, a homonymous superior quadrantanopia, and alexia without agraphia. Smaller infarcts localized to the anterior, midline, or mediodorsal nuclei of the thalamus may cause an isolated amnestic syndrome or anomia. Alexia without agraphia has been reported with infarcts of the left lingual gyrus with or without involvement of the splenium of the corpus callosum.

Memories are formed in the frontal lobes, basal forebrain, thalami, and mesial temporal lobes by connections as described by Papez. Amnesia is a pervasive impairment of the ability to recall and recognize unique events and unique stimuli. Retrograde amnesia is amnesia for information learned before the onset of the illness. Anterograde amnesia is amnesia for information that should have been acquired after onset of illness. The etiologies of amnesia are myriad. Amnestic syndromes of sudden onset (Table 26.1) usually show gradual but incomplete recovery.

Some amnestic syndromes occur suddenly but are transitory, including those seen with partial complex seizures, postconcussive states, and transient global amnesia. Amnestic syndromes of subacute onset as seen in patients with Wernicke-Korsakoff syndrome, herpes simplex encephalitis, tuberculosis, and other basilar meningitides,

> ## TABLE 26.1: AMNESTIC SYNDROMES WITH SUDDEN ONSET
>
> ▓ Bilateral hippocampal infarction due to atheroembolic occlusive disease of the posterior cerbral arteries or their inferior temporal branches
> ▓ Trauma to the diencephalic or inferomedial temporal regions
> ▓ Spontaneous subarachnoid hemorrhage
> ▓ Carbon monoxide and other hypoxic states

have varying degrees of recovery and usually leave sequelae. Slowly progressive amnestic states may be caused by tumors involving the floor and walls of the third ventricle or Alzheimer disease or other degenerative dementias.

■ SELECTED REFERENCES

Benson DF, Marsden CD, Meadows JC. The amnesic syndrome of posterior cerebral artery occlusion. *Acta Neurologica Scandinavica* 1974;50:133–145.

De Renzi E, Zambolin A, Crisi G. The pattern of neuro-psychological impairment associated with left posterior cerebral artery infarcts. *Brain* 1987;110:1099–1116.

Ott BR, Saver JL. Unilateral amnesic stroke. Six new cases and a review of the literature. *Stroke* 1993;24:1033–1042.

Papez JW. A proposed mechanism of emotion. *Arch Neurol Pathol* 1937;38:725–743.

■ SEE QUESTIONS: 49, 115, 164

CASE 27

DEMENTIA (EARLY ALZHEIMER DISEASE)

OBJECTIVES

▓ To discuss the diagnosis of dementia.
▓ To discuss the diagnosis of Alzheimer disease.
▓ To discuss the treatment of Alzheimer disease.

VIGNETTE

A 75-year-old man had memory problems over the past 12 months.

CASE SUMMARY

This 75-year-old man noted he was having difficulty with his short-term memory. His wife noted difficulty doing simple calculations and remembering recent conversations. On one occasion while staying in an unfamiliar environment, he was confused, unclothed, and was trying to enter the hotel rooms of others. His past medical history is notable for pulmonary fibrosis and hyperlipidemia but he has no history of previous stroke, significant head trauma, or CNS infection. He does not drink alcohol excessively and is on no medications that would obviously affect his cognition. He has no family history of dementia.

His examination shows that he is oriented to person, place, and time except that he has difficulty naming the month. Immediate recall and attention appear unremarkable. He was able to name two of three objects on testing short-term recall. He was not obviously aphasic, was able to follow multistep commands, and had no construction apraxia on bedside testing. He was begun on galantamine for a diagnosis of early Alzheimer disease.

Dementia is defined as a decline in memory and at least one other cognitive function (aphasia, apraxia, agnosia, decline in executive function) that impairs social or occupational functioning. Dementia has many causes including degenerative, vascular, infectious, psychiatric (especially depression), toxic, metabolic, traumatic, and brain structural etiologies. Most of the nondegenerative causes can be excluded with appropriate history (especially medications), general and neurologic examination, head imaging study, and laboratory evaluation. Neuropsychologic testing is done to define the specific cognitive abnormalities, which often follow a pattern consistent with a specific diagnosis.

The most common causes of dementia are Alzheimer disease and vascular dementia. The second and third most common degenerative dementias are Lewy body disease and the frontotemporal dementias. Definitive Alzheimer disease is diagnosed only in those patients with a clinical syndrome consistent with it and histopathologic confirmation based on biopsy or autopsy brain specimens. Alzheimer disease is diagnosed clinically when there is gradual and progressive decline or impairment of recent memory and one other aspect of cognition; the cognitive deficits are not due to other psychiatric, neurologic, or systemic diseases; and the deficits do not occur exclusively in the setting of delirium. The Mini-Mental State Exam (MMSE) is a common bedside test for dementia. It tests a range of cognitive functions including orientation, recall, attention, calculation, language function, and constructional praxis. The total maximum score is 30.

The treatment of dementia is directed at the underlying cause, especially if it is a potentially reversible cause. Symptomatic treatment is available for Alzheimer disease. Three acetylcholinesterase inhibitor medications (donepezil, rivastigmine, galantamine) are available that slow the progression of Alzheimer disease, and some patients may show an improvement in cognition initially. In addition, the N-methyl-D aspartate receptor antagonist (NMDA) memanitine, has been recently approved for treatment of moderate- to severe Alzheimer disease. Vitamin E supplementation may also by useful in Alzheimer disease. Medications are often used to control some of the behavioral symptoms noted in demented patients.

■ SELECTED REFERENCES

Biller J, ed. *Practical neurology,* 2nd ed. Philadelphia: Lippincott Williams & Wilkins, 2002.

Knopman DS, DeKosky ST, Cummings JL, et al. Practice parameter: diagnosis of dementia (an evidence-based review). Report of the Quality Standards Subcommittee of the American Academy of Neurology. *Neurology* 2001;56:1143–1153.

■ SEE QUESTIONS: 86, 106, 107, 109, 110

CASE 28

DEMENTIA (LATE ALZHEIMER DISEASE)

OBJECTIVES

- To discuss the diagnosis of dementia.
- To discuss the treatment of Alzheimer disease.
- To discuss the treatment of the behavioral manifestations of Alzheimer disease.

VIGNETTE

An 85-year-old man had a 3-year history of gradually progressive memory loss.

CASE SUMMARY

This 85-year-old man has had a progressive memory loss for 2 to 3 years. His wife was having some trouble caring for him and was concerned he might wander out of the house, which he had done in the past. He had a history of a right middle cerebral artery infarction (frontal lobe) secondary to a right internal carotid artery occlusion. He also had a history of a bilateral postural hand tremor. He was initially begun on donepezil and vitamin E supplementation. His donepezil was discontinued as his wife did not feel it was effective. He was also prescribed low-dose levetiracetam for probable multifocal myoclonus. For mild depression he was prescribed mirtazapine and later tried escitalopram. He was later prescribed rivastigmine for his dementia.

His examination showed his disorientation to time and place, poor immediate and short-term recall, poor simple calculation, difficulty following multistep commands, and trouble with writing a sentence and copying a figure. His answers were hesitant and at times he perseverated when responding. He had a neuropsychological examination performed between the periods of taking cholinesterase inhibitors. He showed significant problems with orientation and very poor short-term recall and recall of recent events. His recognition memory was notably impaired as was his semantic fluency and confrontation naming. He scored a 13/30 on the Mini-Mental State Exam. He had marked subjective depression on the Geriatric Depression Inventory. It was thought he had a generalized dementia of moderate severity that was greater than expected for his previous stroke.

Dementia is defined as a decline in memory and at least one other cognitive function (aphasia, apraxia, agnosia, decline in executive function) that impairs social or occupational functioning. Dementia has many causes including degenerative, vascular, infectious, psychiatric (especially depression), toxic, metabolic, traumatic, and brain structural etiologies. Most of the nondegenerative causes can be excluded with appropriate history (especially medications), general and neurologic examination, head imaging study, and laboratory evaluation. Neuropsychologic testing is done to define the specific cognitive abnormalities, which often follow a pattern consistent with a specific diagnosis.

The most common causes of dementia are Alzheimer disease and vascular dementia. As demonstrated by his wife's concern for his safety, caring for patients with Alzheimer disease can be quite demanding. Often in the later stages patients can be agitated, anxious, depressed, and have sleep disorders. Hallucinations and delusions as well as bizarre or violent behavior can occur. Impaired judgment and wandering are especially challenging because of patient safety issues.

Symptomatic treatment is available for Alzheimer disease. Three acetylcholinesterase inhibitor medications (donepezil, rivastigmine, galantamine) are available that slow the progression of Alzheimer disease, and some patients may show an improvement in cognition initially. In addition, the N-methyl-D aspartate receptor antagonist (NMDA) memanitine, has been recently approved for treatment of moderate- to severe Alzheimer disease. Vitamin E supplementation may also be useful in Alzheimer disease. Medications are often used to control some of the behavioral symptoms noted in demented patients. Atypical neuroleptic agents can be used for agitation, hallucinations, delusions, and unusual behaviors. Selective serotonin reuptake inhibitors seem to work well for depression and are fairly well tolerated. Anxiety and excessive motor activities may respond to the atypical neuroleptic agents or low doses of benzodiazepines. In general, all medications should be started at low doses and increased slowly.

■ SELECTED REFERENCES

Biller J, ed. *Practical neurology,* 2nd ed. Philadelphia: Lippincott Williams & Wilkins, 2002.

Knopman DS, DeKosky ST, Cummings JL, et al. Practice parameter: diagnosis of dementia (an evidence-based review). Report of the Quality Standards Subcommittee of the American Academy of Neurology. *Neurology* 2001;56:1143–1153.

■ SEE QUESTIONS: 86, 106, 107, 109, 110, 174

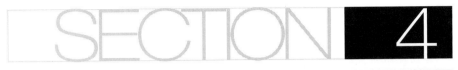

SECTION 4

CEREBROVASCULAR

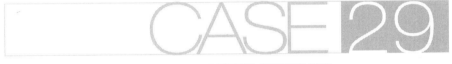

CASE 29

ASYMPTOMATIC CAROTID ARTERY STENOSIS

OBJECTIVES

- To review the epidemiology of asymptomatic carotid artery bruits and stenosis.
- To review our current understanding on the management of patients with asymptomatic carotid artery stenosis.

VIGNETTE

A 67-year-old man with a history of diabetes, hypertension, and coronary artery disease was found to have a left carotid bruit. He had no retinal or hemispheric ischemic events.

CASE SUMMARY

Our patient was found to have an asymptomatic carotid bruit, and subsequent non-invasive studies (carotid ultrasound and MRA) showed an underlying 50% to 79% carotid artery stenosis. Asymptomatic carotid artery atherosclerosis is highly prevalent in the general population, particularly in the elderly. Compared with symptomatic carotid artery stenosis, asymptomatic carotid artery stenosis is associated with a relatively low risk of ipsilateral cerebral infarction. About 4% of adults have asymptomatic neck bruits, but a carotid bruit is a poor predictor of extracranial carotid artery disease or high-grade carotid artery stenosis.

Persons with asymptomatic carotid bruits have an estimated annual risk of stroke of 1.5% at 1 year and 7.5% at 5 years. Asymptomatic carotid artery stenosis of 75%

or less carries a stroke risk of 1.3% annually. When the carotid artery stenosis is more than 75%, the combined rate for TIA and stroke is 10.5% per year, with most events occurring ipsilateral to the stenosed carotid artery.

Data from five randomized clinical trials on the efficacy of carotid endarterectomy (CEA) in patients with asymptomatic carotid artery stenosis are now available. The study by Clagget and colleagues concluded that most asymptomatic patients with cervical bruits and abnormal pneumoplethysmography are appropriately managed without surgery. The Carotid Artery Surgery Asymptomatic Narrowing Operation Versus Aspirin (CASANOVA) trial included asymptomatic patients with carotid artery stenosis of 50% to 90%. Patients with more than 90% stenosis were excluded on the basis of presumed surgical benefit. All patients were treated with 330 mg of aspirin and 75 mg of dipyridamole three times daily. Overall, the trial showed no difference between medically and surgically treated groups.

The Mayo Asymptomatic Carotid Endarterectomy (MACE) trial was terminated early because of a significantly higher number of myocardial infarctions and TIAs in the surgical group. The results most likely reflected the avoidance of aspirin in the surgical group.

The Veterans Affairs Asymptomatic Carotid Endarterectomy Trial compared the outcomes of surgery and medical treatment among 444 asymptomatic patients with angiographically proven carotid artery stenosis of 50% to 99%. The study results showed a reduction in the relative risk of ipsilateral neurological events with surgery when TIAs and stroke were included as composite endpoints. However, when ipsilateral stroke was considered alone, only a nonsignificant trend favoring surgery was noted. For the combined outcome of stroke and death, no significant differences were found between the two treatment arms.

The Asymptomatic Carotid Atherosclerosis Study (ACAS) compared the use of carotid endarterectomy, aspirin therapy, and medical risk factor management in patients younger than 80 years who had asymptomatic carotid artery stenosis of 60% or more. The degree of stenosis was determined by arteriography, by Doppler ultrasound scanning within 60 days (greater than 95% positive predictive value by frequency or flow velocity), or, in a separate study, by Doppler ultrasound scanning performed within 60 days and confirmed by oculopneumoplethysmography (more than 90% positive predictive value). The angiographic methods were similar to those used in the North American Symptomatic Carotid Endarectomy Trial (NASCET).

Based on a 5-year projection, the ACAS showed that carotid endarterectomy reduced the absolute risk of stroke by 5.9% (which corresponds to an absolute risk reduction of only 1.2% per year) and the relative risk of stroke and death by 53%. The surgical benefit incorporated a low aggregate perioperative stroke and death rate of only 2.3%, including a permanent arteriographic complication rate of 1.2%.

Despite the ACAS findings, some investigators still feel that insufficient evidence exists to recommend surgery in asymptomatic patients. Because of the low risk of stroke in asymptomatic patients, some experts recommend surgery only when the degree of stenosis is more than 80%, provided that the operation is performed by an experienced surgeon with a complication rate of 3% or less.

■ SELECTED REFERENCES

Biller J, Thies WH. Carotid endarterectomy is warranted in selected symptomatic patients. *Am Fam Phys* 2000;61:400–406.

Fleck JD, Biller J. Choices in medical management for prevention of acute ischemic stroke. *Curr Neurol Neurosci Rep* 2001:1(Jan)33–38.

■ SEE QUESTIONS: 32, 89, 93

CASE 30

VERTEBROBASILAR TIAs: BASILAR ARTERY STENOSIS

OBJECTIVES

- To review the clinical manifestations of TIAs in the vertebrobasilar circulation.
- To review the clinical manifestations of TIAs in the carotid circulation.
- To review therapeutic strategies for symptomatic basilar artery stenosis.

VIGNETTE

A 78-year-old hypertensive man was evaluated because of a 12-month history of recurrent brief nonpositional spells of slurred speech, double vision, circumoral numbness, left-sided weakness, and loss of balance. The patient received platelet antiaggregants and more recently was treated with warfarin without resolution of his spells.

CASE SUMMARY

Atherosclerosis of the major intracranial arteries is an important cause of ischemic stroke, especially among African-Americans and Asians. Our patient had recurrent episodes of vertebrobasilar ischemia, associated with a high grade basilar artery stenosis. He underwent angioplasty and stenting of the basilar artery, as he experienced disabling refractory episodes of vertebrobasilar ischemia, despite the use of several antiplatelet agents alone or in combination and the use of warfarin.

The brainstem, cerebellum, and labyrinths are supplied by the vertebrobasilar arterial system. The basilar artery is formed by the vertebral arteries at the level of the pontomedullary junction. The artery has three branches on each side that provide the blood supply to the cerebellum. The posterior inferior cerebellar artery (PICA) usually originates from the vertebral artery, whereas the anterior inferior

TABLE 30.1: CLINICOANATOMICAL CORRELATION OF DISORDERS OF NEUROVASCULAR FUNCTION

	Neurovascular Cerebral		Cranial Nerves	Motorl Reflexes Cerebellari Gait	Sensory
Carotid TIA	Carotid bruit, decreased carotid pulse	Transient aphasia and dysaarthria	Ipsilateral amaurosis fugax, contralateral HH	Transient contralateral weakness or clumsiness	Transient contralateral loss
Vertebro basilar TIA	Vertebral or basilar bruit	Normal	Transient CN findings— diplopia, dysarthria	Transient bilateral weakness or clumsiness	Transient bilateral loss

HH, homonymous hemianopia.

cerebellar artery (AICA) and the superior cerebellar artery (SCA) arise from the basilar artery.

A *transient ischemic attack* (TIA) is a transient episode of focal neurological or retinal dysfunction of acute onset secondary to impaired blood supply in a vascular territory. The attacks last less than 24 hours leaving no residual deficits. Because the episodes usually last less than 20 minutes, patients often have no clinical manifestations by the time they present to medical attention. Clinical signs typical of TIAs in the carotid and vertebrobasilar territories are outlined in Table 30.1. It should be noted that transient vertigo, diplopia, dysarthria, or dysphagia in isolation is insufficient to establish a diagnosis of vertebrobasilar TIAs (Table 30.2).

In addition, isolated drop attacks in which the patient falls to the ground, maintains consciousness, and then arises without a deficit are seldom due to vertebrobasilar

TABLE 30.2: SYMPTOMS SUGGESTIVE OF VERTEBROBASILAR TRANSIENT ISCHEMIC ATTACKS

- Usually bilateral weakness or clumsiness, but may be unilateral or shifting
- Bilateral, shifting, or crossed (ipsilateral face and contralateral body) sensory loss or paresthesias
- Bilateral or contralateral homonymous visual field defects or binocular vision loss
- Two or more of the following symptoms: vertigo, diplopia, dysphagia, dysarthria, and ataxia
- Symptoms not acceptable as evidence of transient ischemic attack:
  - Syncope, dizziness, confusion, urinary or fecal incontinence, and generalized weakness
  - Isolated occurrence of vertigo, diplopia, dysphagia, ataxia, tinnitus, amnesia, drop attacks, or dysarthria

ischemia. The recognition of TIAs is important, because 10% to 30% of patients with ischemic stroke, some of which may have been preventable, have a history of earlier TIAs. The annual risk of stroke after a TIA is 3% to 4% per year. However, the risk of a subsequent stroke is at least three times greater for individuals who have had a TIA than in those individuals who have not had a TIA.

Within the past few years, carotid artery angioplasty and stenting (CAS) placement have evolved as an alternative treatment for extracranial carotid artery disease. Recent studies also suggest that intracranial angioplasty and stenting are promising therapies for patients with symptomatic intracranial arterial stenosis. Vertebrobasilar and intracranial angioplasty have also been attempted with a good degree of technical safety and with promising results in selected cases. Fear of distal embolization and stroke during the procedure continues to arouse concerns.

■ SELECTED REFERENCES

Chimowitz MI. Angioplasty or stenting is not appropriate as first line treatment of intracranial stenosis. *Arch Neurol* 2001;58:1690–1692.

Fernandez-Beer E, Biller J. Cerebrovascular disorders. *Curr Pract Med* 1999;2:745–752.

Lutsep HL, Barnwell SL, Mawad M, et al. Stenting of symptomatic atherosclerotic lesions in the vertebral or intracranial arteries (SSYLVIA): study results. *Stroke* 2003;34:253(abst).

Marks MP, Marcellus M, Norbash AM, et al. Outcome of angioplasty for atherosclerotic intracranial stenosis. *Stroke* 1999;30:1065–1069.

■ SEE QUESTIONS: 46, 47, 49, 50, 64, 65

CASE 31

DYSPHAGIA/IMBALANCE: VERTEBRAL ARTERY STENOSIS

OBJECTIVES

- To review the important morbidity associated with dysphagia.
- To discuss the different pathogenetic mechanisms of dysphagia and dysarthria.
- To illustrate the potential risks of catheter cerebral angiography.

VIGNETTE

A 71-year-old man with a history of CABG, left carotid endarterectomy, abdominal aortic aneurysm (AAA) repair, bilateral femoral artery bypass, hypertension, and cigarette smoking was evaluated because of a 9-month history of slurred speech, swallowing difficulties, and tongue weakness. He also had headaches and posterior neck pain and once he had a "passing out spell"; since that event, he has experienced balance difficulties.

CASE SUMMARY

Disorders of swallowing and articulation can be acute, subacute, chronic, persistent, or episodic and can be caused by a variety of central nervous system and peripheral neuromuscular diseases. Our patient had multiple vascular risk factors, including arterial hypertension and cigarette smoking. He had a prior coronary artery bypass graft, abdominal aortic aneurysm repair, and aortofemoral artery bypass surgery. He consulted us because of subacute progressive and persistent swallowing and speech difficulties, imbalance, and posterior neck pain. Other symptoms of vertebrobasilar ischemia such as dizziness, vertigo, diplopia, perioral numbness, alternating paresthesias, drop attacks, and homonymous visual field defects were lacking.

Although he had an apparent "passing out spell," this was not typical for syncope due to glossopharyngeal or vagal dysfunction. The most worrisome complaint was his oropharyngeal dysphagia. He had no evidence of hoarseness. The dysphagia caused him to have considerable weight loss. His examination was remarkable for dysarthria, hypernasal voice, impaired tongue movements, asymmetric and brisk lower extremity muscle stretch reflexes, and a left Babinski sign. He had no emotional incontinence and his gait was normal. He had no evidence of muscle atrophy nor muscle weakness or fasciculations.

Early identification and systematic evaluation of dysphagia or difficulty with swallowing is important. In particular, elderly patients with dysphagia have a high risk of aspiration pneumonia. Furthermore, dysphagia is also of concern because of its potential for malnutrition, dehydration, and airway obstruction. Because bedside dysphagia testing is not reliable at detecting silent aspiration, fiberoptic evaluation or fluoroscopic examination is recommended for severe dysphagia.

In our patient, ancillary investigations showed no evidence of muscle or neuromuscular junction abnormalities or motor neuron disease. There was no evidence of multiple cranial neuropathies or basal ganglia disease. He had no evidence of intrinsic brainstem lesions at the level of the glossopharyngeal and vagus nerves, but rather a slight extrinsic encroachment of the medulla by what later on proved to be atherosclerotic tortuosity and elongation involving the vertebrobasilar arterial system.

The vertebrobasilar circulation supplies blood to the brainstem, cerebellum, and occipital lobes via the paired vertebral arteries, which converge to form the basilar artery at the pontomedullary junction. Atherothrombotic disease in the vertebrobasilar system has a predilection for the distal vertebral artery and the lower or middle basilar artery. Catheter cerebral angiography is an invasive investigation with an overall combined minor and major complication (primarily stroke) rate of approximately 1.0%. Our patient had a small cerebellar and occipital lobe infarction following catheter cerebral angiography. Fortunately, he had a complete neurological recovery.

■ **SELECTED REFERENCES**

Biller J, ed. *Practical neurology,* 2nd ed. Philadelphia: Lippincott Williams & Wilkins, 2002.
Dray TG, Hillel AD, Miller RM. Dysphagia caused by neurological deficits. *Otolaryngol Clin North Am* 1998;31:507–523.
Hankey GJ, Warlow CP, Molyneous AJ. Complications of cerebral angiography for patients with mild carotid territory ischaemia being considered for carotid endarterectomy. *J Neurol Neurosurg Psychiatry* 1990;53:542–548.
Ramsey DJ, Smithard DG, Kalra L. Early assessment of dysphagia and aspiration risk in acute stroke patients. *Stroke* 2003;34:1252–1257.

■ **SEE QUESTION: 50**

CASE 32

PURE MOTOR HEMIPARESIS DUE TO CAPSULAR LACUNAR INFARCTION

OBJECTIVES

▤ To review the clinical characteristics of the most common lacunar syndrome, pure motor hemiparesis.
▤ To discuss the importance of careful follow-up of patients with lacunar stroke.
▤ To review risk factors for stroke recurrence.

VIGNETTE

In May 1998, this 82-year-old left-handed woman with a history of hypertension and hyperlipidemia complained of a sudden onset of right-sided weakness and slurred speech. On admission, she was also found to have an inferior wall myocardial infarction.

CASE SUMMARY

Ischemic stroke encompasses a range of pathogenetic mechanisms including large artery atherosclerotic disease with artery-to-artery embolism, cardioembolism, small vessel disease (lacunar) stroke, and stroke of undetermined cause. Approximately 20% of strokes are due to lacunar infarctions. The risk of recurrent stroke is lowest for lacunar strokes. The overall stroke recurrence rate among patients with lacunar infarctions within 3 months has been estimated to be 1.2%. Patients with a lacunar stroke index event are equally likely to have recurrent small and large vessel ischemic strokes.

Our patient had a pure motor hemiparesis caused by an internal capsule lacunar infarction. She initially received prophylactic antiplatelet therapy. She then developed atrial fibrillation and received treatment with warfarin. Nonvalvular atrial fibrillation increases the risk for stroke sixfold. Warfarin therapy reduces the rate of stroke by 68% [95% confidence interval (CI), 50% to 79%], and aspirin reduces the rate of stroke by 21%. When balanced against the risk for major hemorrhage (1.3% for warfarin, 1.0% per year for aspirin), warfarin therapy was justified in our patient. She subsequently required a pacemaker due to a high-degree atrioventricular (AV) block.

Pure motor hemiparesis is the most common lacunar syndrome and may also be caused by a basis pontis or corona radiata lacuna. Pure motor hemiparesis is characterized by contralateral hemiparesis or hemiplegia involving the face, arm, and to a lesser extent, the leg, accompanied by mild dysarthria, particularly at onset of stroke. There should be no aphasia, apraxia, or agnosia, and there are no sensory, visual, or other higher cortical disturbances. Headache and seizures do not occur with lacunar infarctions. Multiple lacunar infarctions may cause a pseudobulbar syndrome.

■ SELECTED REFERENCES

Biller J, ed. *Practical neurology,* 2nd ed. Philadelphia: Lippincott Williams & Wilkins, 2002.

Brazis PW, Masdeu JC, Biller J. *Localization in clinical neurology,* 4th ed. Philadelphia: Lippincott Williams & Wilkins, 2001.

Kappelle LJ, van Latum JC, van Swieten JC, et al. Recurrent stroke after transient ischemic attack or minor ischaemic stroke: does the distinction between small and large vessel disease remain true to type? Dutch TIA Trial Study Group. *J Neurol Neurosurg Psychiatry* 1995;64:771–776.

Moroney JT, Bagiella E, Paik MC, et al. Risk factors for early recurrence after ischemic stroke: the role of stroke syndrome and subtype. *Stroke* 1998;29:2118–2124.

■ SEE QUESTIONS: 32, 36, 70, 87, 88, 95, 148, 149, 167, 233

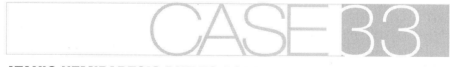

ATAXIC HEMIPARESIS DUE TO PONTINE INFARCTION

OBJECTIVES

- To describe the clinical characteristics of ataxic hemiparesis (homolateral ataxia and crural paresis).
- To review the pathogenesis of lacunar infarcts.

▓ To highlight the variety of localizations that can be responsible for ataxic hemiparesis (homolateral ataxia and crural paresis).
▓ To review variants of this syndrome.

VIGNETTE

A 75-year-old woman with a history of hypertension and hyperlipidemia had sudden
onset dizziness followed by slurred speech and right-sided weakness.

CASE SUMMARY

Every year at least 750,000 Americans experience a new or recurrent stroke. Cerebrovascular disorders are the result of either ischemia or hemorrhage within the central nervous system (CNS) and are broadly considered under the term *stroke*. Ischemic
strokes resulting from small vessel or penetrating artery disease (lacunes) have unique
clinical, radiological, and pathological features. Lacunar infarcts are small ischemic
infarctions in the deep regions of the brain or brainstem that range in diameter from
0.5 to 15.0 mm. These infarctions result from occlusion of the penetrating arteries,
chiefly the anterior choroidal, middle cerebral, posterior cerebral, and basilar arteries. Lacunar infarcts could also be the result of occlusion of penetrating arteries by
atherosclerosis of the parent artery or by microembolism.

Lacunar syndromes are highly predictive of lacunar infarcts. While there are well
over twenty described lacunar syndromes, the five that have been best described
include pure motor hemiparesis, pure sensory stroke, sensory-motor stroke,
dysarthria–clumsy hand syndrome, and ataxic hemiparesis (homolateral ataxia and
crural paresis). These lacunar syndromes have been described with ischemic lacunar
infarctions as well as with discrete hemorrhages.

Ataxic hemiparesis (homolateral ataxia and crural paresis) is often due to a lacune
affecting either the contralateral posterior limb of the internal capsule or, as in our
patient, the contralateral basis pontis. This syndrome has also been described with
contralateral thalamocapsular lesions, lesions of the contralateral red nucleus, lesions
of the coronal radiata, lentiform nucleus, with superior cerebellar artery territory
infarcts, and with superficial anterior cerebral artery territory infarcts involving the
paracentral region.

Ataxic hemiparesis is characterized by mild to moderate hemiparesis, predominantly involving the lower extremity, and an ipsilateral cerebellar type of incoordination of the arm and leg out of proportion to the weakness. There is usually an extensor
plantar response (Babinski sign) and no evidence of dysarthria. Facial involvement is
rare. Cortical signs or visual field deficits are absent.

Numerous reports have expanded the spectrum of clinical syndromes and signs
associated with ataxic hemiparesis. Included are the hemiataxia-hypesthesia syndrome, painful ataxic hemiparesis, hypesthetic ataxic hemiparesis, ataxic hemiparesis
accompanied by contralateral sensorimotor or motor trigeminal weakness, dysarthia
hemiataxia, and quadrataxic hemiataxia.

■ SELECTED REFERENCES

Biller J, ed. *Practical neurology,* 2nd ed. Philadelphia: Lippincott Willaims & Wilkins, 2002.
Brazis PW, Masdeu JC, Biller J. *Localization in clinical neurology,* 4th ed. Philadelphia: Lippincott Williams & Wilkins, 2001.

■ SEE QUESTIONS: 30, 88, 95, 148, 149, 167

CASE 34

LEFT INTERNAL CAROTID ARTERY DISSECTION

OBJECTIVES

▦ To review the clinical manifestations of extracranial internal carotid artery dissections.
▦ To briefly discuss the pathophysiology of cervicocephalic arterial dissections.
▦ To review common associations predisposing to cervicocephalic arterial dissections.
▦ To analyze current ancillary tests used in the evaluation of cervicocephalic arterial dissections.
▦ To discuss management strategies for patients with extracranial internal carotid artery dissections.

VIGNETTE

A 45-year-old man was sitting at his desk when he suddenly had a sensation of disorientation. This was followed by inability to talk and right-sided weakness. At the same time he noticed a scotoma in the visual field of his left eye. Visual acuity was 20/20-1 OD, 20/70-3 OS. The pinhole test did not increase acuity. There was a partial right inferior homonymous hemianopia. In addition, in both eyes there appeared to be paracentral scotomas in the left field. The pupils were 7 mm in diameter with normal reactions and no relative afferent pupillary defect (RAPD).

CASE SUMMARY

Our patient had a spontaneous left extracranial internal carotid artery dissection leading to left hemispheric and left retinal ischemia, which was successfully treated with intraarterial thrombolysis.

Cervicocephalic arterial dissections are an important cause of stroke in young adults. A dissection is produced by subintimal penetration of blood in a cervicocephalic vessel with subsequent longitudinal extension of the intramural hematoma between its layers. The extracranial internal carotid artery is the site of most dissections. Vertebrobasilar and intracranial carotid artery dissections are less common. Intracranial dissections are usually subintimal and may cause subarachnoid hemorrhage. Multivessel cervicocephalic arterial dissections are a rare occurrence. The recurrence rate of cervicocephalic arterial dissections is approximately 1% per year. The risk of recurrent dissections is higher in young patients and in those with a family history of arterial dissections.

Cervicocephalic arterial dissections often are spontaneous. However, they have been reported after blunt or penetrating trauma and chiropractic manipulation. Intraoral and peritonsillar trauma is an important cause in children. The trauma itself may be trivial. They have also been associated with fibromuscular dysplasia, Marfan syndrome, Ehlers-Danlos syndrome type IV, pseudoxanthoma elasticum, Menkes disease, osteogenesis imperfecta Type I, coarctation of the aorta, adult polycystic kidney disease, cystic medial necrosis, reticular fiber deficiency, accumulation of mucopolysaccharides, elevated arterial elastase content, atherosclerosis, extreme vessel tortuosity, Moyamoya disease, homocystinuria, pharyngeal infections, luetic arteritis, α_1 antitrypsin deficiency, sympathomimetic drug abuse, and lentiginosis.

Cervicocephalic arterial dissections should be considered in the differential diagnosis of TIAs or cerebral infarction in any young adult, particularly when traditional vascular risk factors are missing. Other signs and symptoms associated with extracranial internal carotid artery dissections may also include hemicranial headaches plus a Horner's syndrome; an isolated Horner's syndrome; hemicranial headaches plus delayed hemispheric or retinal ischemia; head, orbital, face, or neck pain; scalp tenderness; scintillations; subjective audible bruit; tinnitus; light-headedeness or syncope; and cranial nerve palsies. In addition to a postganglionic Horner's syndrome, neuroophthalmological manifestations of internal carotid artery dissections may also include central or branch retinal artery occlusion, ophthalmic artery occlusion, ischemic optic neuropathy, homonymous hemianopia, and ocular motor nerve palsies CN III, IV, and VI. A postganglionic Horner's syndrome results in facial anhidrosis.

The diagnosis of cervicocephalic arterial dissection is often based on arteriographic findings. Arteriographic features include the presence of a pearl and string sign; double lumen sign; short, smooth, tapered occlusion; or pseudoanueyrsm formation. High-resolution magnetic resonance imaging (MRI), magnetic resonance angiography (MRA), and ultrafast spiral CT (3D CT angiography) provide valuable noninvasive information and are increasingly replacing catheter angiography. MRI demonstrates the intramural hematoma and the false lumen of the dissected artery. Ultrasound studies can be helpful in monitoring the course and treatment of the disease.

Treatment of cervicocephalic arterial dissections includes anticoagulation with intravenous unfractionated heparin followed by 3 to 6 months of warfarin. Platelet antiaggregants are used by many physicians because of the lack of solid data for the use of anticoagulants. Anticoagulation should be withheld in patients with intracranial dissections (particularly involving the vertebrobasilar circulation) because of the risk of subarachnoid hemorrhage. A cervicocephalic arterial dissection is not a contraindication for the use of thrombolytics, if no other exclusions exist. Surgical correction has been used in selected patients who have not responded to medical therapy. Stents have been used in selected patients.

■ SELECTED REFERENCES

Biller J, ed. *Practical neurology,* 2nd ed. Philadelphia: Lippincott Williams & Wilkins, 2002.
Love BB, Biller J. Stroke in young adults. In: Samuels MA, Keske SF, eds. *Office practice of neurology,* 2nd ed. New York: Churchill Livingstone, 2003:337–358.

■ SEE QUESTIONS: 29, 43, 44, 45, 46, 70, 89, 95, 112, 167, 233

CASE 35

WALLENBERG SYNDROME SECONDARY TO VERTEBRAL ARTERY DISSECTION

OBJECTIVES

▓ To review the clinical manifestations of the lateral medullary syndrome (Wallenberg syndrome).
▓ To briefly discuss the clinical manifestations of vertebrobasilar dissections.
▓ To review common associations predisposing to vertebrobasilar dissections.

VIGNETTE

A 33-year-old man presented to an ER with sudden onset of severe posterior neck pain, dizziness, unsteadiness, nausea, and vomiting. A head CT was performed, which was normal. He is a block mason whose work involves heavy lifting.

CASE SUMMARY

Our patient had classical symptoms and signs of a lateral medullary syndrome (Wallenberg syndrome) due to a vertebral artery dissection. Wallenberg syndrome is most often caused by occlusion of the intracranial segment of the vertebral artery. Less commonly it is caused by an occlusion of the posterior inferior cerebellar (PICA) artery. This syndrome produces an ipsilateral Horner syndrome; loss of pain and temperature sensation in the face; weakness of the palate, pharynx, and vocal cords;

and cerebellar ataxia. Contralateral to the lesion, there is hemibody loss of pain and temperature sensation.

Vertebrobasilar artery dissection due to cervical trauma, vigorous gymnastics, and chiropractic manipulation of the cervical spine is an underrecognized etiology of stroke in young adults and children. Signs and symptoms associated with vertebrobasilar dissections include occipital or posterior neck pain, mastoid pain, vertebrobasilar transient ischemic attacks, variations of the lateral or medial medullary infarction, cerebellar infarction, and posterior cerebral artery distribution infarction.

■ SELECTED REFERENCES

Brazis PW, Masdeu JC, Biller J. *Practical neurology,* 4th ed. Philadelphia: Lippincott Williams & Wilkins, 2001.
Love BB, Biller J. Stroke in young adults. In: Samuels MA, Keske SF, eds. *Office practice of neurology,* 2nd ed. New York: Churchill Livingstone, 2003:337–358.

■ SEE QUESTIONS: 19, 35, 36, 38, 95

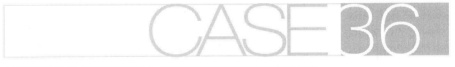

MULTIPLE CEREBRAL INFARCTIONS DUE TO ANTIPHOSPHOLIPID ANTIBODY SYNDROME

OBJECTIVES

■ To review the main manifestations of the antiphospholipid antibody syndrome (APAS).
■ To discuss nosological entities associated with the secondary type of APAS.
■ To summarize therapeutic guidelines for arterial thrombosis associated with APAS.

VIGNETTE

In October 1992, this 45-year-old woman, with a history of pregnancy-induced hypertension (HTN) and preeclampsia, had her first stroke, affecting her left hemibody. The patient received warfarin. In August 1994, while on warfarin, she lost consciousness and was diagnosed with acute obstructive hydrocephalus secondary to a pineal gland hemorrhage. A ventriculoperitoneal (VP) shunt was placed. In 1995, she had two hemispheric strokes. The patient received aspirin. On December 25, 2002, she had an episode of vomiting, diarrhea, right-hand weakness, and trouble speaking. The patient was treated with aspirin and dipyridamole.

CASE SUMMARY

The patient's history is consistent with an antiphospholipid antibody syndrome (APAS). Lupus anticoagulant and anticardiolipin antibodies are known collectively as antiphospholipid antibodies. Antiphospholipid antibodies are a recognized cause of recurrent arterial and venous thromboembolism. Ischemic stroke is the most common arterial thrombotic event in APAS. APAS associates the presence of antiphospholipid antibodies in high titers with recurrent arterial or venous thromboses, fetal loss, and livedo reticularis.

Several antiphospholipid antibodies have been described in IgG, IgA, or IgM isotypes: anticardiolipin (aCL), antiphosphatidylethanolamine (aPE), antiphosphatidylserine (aPS), and antiphosphatidylcholine (aPC). The component required for aCL binding is β_2-glycoprotein 1.

APAS may be primary or secondary to underlying diseases such as systemic lupus erythematosus (SLE), rheumatoid arthritis, Sjögren's syndrome, Sneddon's syndrome (livedo reticularis and ischemic cerebrovascular disease), malignancies, syphilis, acute and chronic infections including AIDS, inflammatory bowel disease, administration of certain drugs, liver transplantation, early-onset severe preeclampsia, and also in individuals without demonstrable underlying disorder.

Antiphospholipid antibodies are associated with recurrent fetal loss, thrombocytopenia, a false-positive Venereal Disease Research Laboratories (VDRL) test, livedo reticularis, and may also cause severe thrombosis leading to cerebral and ocular ischemia, myocardial infarction, peripheral arterial thromboembolism, as well as venous thrombosis and pulmonary emboli. Multiple cerebral infarctions (as in our patient) are common in patients with APAS; a subset of patients may present with vascular dementia. Still another group may have an acute ischemic encephalopathy.

Pathological studies of cerebral arteries involved in association with antiphospholipid antibodies demonstrate the presence of a chronic thrombotic microangiopathy, but no evidence of vasculitis. Patients with antiphospholipid antibodies have an increased frequency of mitral and aortic vegetations resembling verrucous endocarditis (Libman-Sacks endocarditis).

Treatment for arterial thrombosis associated with antiphospholipid antibodies is not well established. It is accepted that oral anticoagulation with warfarin is the preferred treatment for the prevention of thromboembolic events in patients with APAS. Warfarin should be replaced by low molecular weight heparin or unfractionated heparin in case of pregnancy. The use of antiplatelet drugs is also reasonable in the prevention of thrombosis in APAS if anticoagulation is contraindicated. Although they have not yet been tested in prospective studies, antimalarial drugs might be useful in APAS patients with or without associated SLE.

■ SELECTED REFERENCES

Biller J, ed. *Practical neurology,* 2nd ed. Philadelphia: Lippincott Williams & Wilkins, 2002.
Cuadrado MJ, Hughes GRV. Antiphospholipid (Hughes) syndrome. *Rheum Dis Clin North Am* 2001;27:507–524.

Levine SR, Welch KMA. The spectrum of neurologic disease associated with antiphospholipid antibodies. Lupus anticoagulants and anticardiolipin antibodies. *Arch Neurol* 1987;44:876–883.

■ **SEE QUESTIONS: 20, 54, 71, 94, 96, 97, 160, 161**

CASE 37

PSEUDOBULBAR PALSY (MULTIPLE STROKES)

OBJECTIVES

▨ To review the clinical characteristics of the syndrome of pseudobulbar palsy.
▨ To discuss the pathogenetic mechanisms of the syndrome of pseudobulbar palsy.
▨ To describe nonvascular etiologies of the syndrome of pseudobulbar palsy.

VIGNETTE

A 48-year-old man with a history of hypertension, cigarette smoking, and prior strokes was admitted for evaluation of progressive difficulty speaking and swallowing. The patient had a greater than 40-pound weight loss over the past year. Additional vascular risk factors included a left atrial appendage thrombus and heterozygosity for factor V Leiden.

CASE SUMMARY

Our patient had multiple vascular risk factors, including arterial hypertension and cigarette smoking. He also had evidence of a left atrial appendage thrombus and was heterozygous for the factor V Leiden mutation. High blood pressure is the most significant risk factor for stroke. If a patient has high blood pressure, the risk of stroke increases four- to sixfold. An estimated 40% to 90% of stroke patients are diagnosed with high blood pressure before their attack. Cigarette smoking nearly doubles the risk for ischemic stroke. The risk of stroke declines significantly in two to four years after quitting, although it takes several decades to return to the risk level of someone who has never smoked. The contribution of the factor V Leiden mutation and the risk for acute cerebral arterial thrombosis is uncertain.

The patient's dysphagia caused him to have considerable weight loss. His examination was remarkable for dysarthria, hypernasal voice, automatic voluntary dissociation of facial movements, primitive reflexes, and asymmetric and brisk muscle stretch reflexes. He also reported emotional incontinence with pathological laughing and crying and had a small-stepped gait (marche à petit pas), all features suggestive of the syndrome of pseudobulbar palsy. In our patient, the pseudobulbar palsy was caused by multiple subcortical infarctions as demonstrated by neuroimaging studies.

Other less common vascular etiologies of pseudobulbar palsy include diverse conditions such as the antiphospholipid antibody syndrome and embolism from atrial myxomas. The syndrome of pseudobulbar palsy has also been associated with a variety of inflammatory, infectious, demyelinative, neoplastic, chemotherapeutic agents (i.e., cytosine arabinoside), amyotrophic lateral sclerosis, and other neuromuscular disorders, and has also been reported after posterior fossa surgery in children.

■ SELECTED REFERENCES

Biller J, ed. *Practical neurology,* 2nd ed. Philadelphia: Lippincott Williams & Wilkins, 2002.
Brazis PW, Masdeu JC, Biller J. *Localization in clinical neurology,* 4th ed. Philadelphia: Lippincott Williams & Wilkins, 2001.
Mancardi GL, Romagnoli P, Tassinari T, et al. Lacunae and cribriform cavities of the brain. Correlations with pseudobulbar palsy and parkinsonism. *Eur Neurol* 1988;28(1):11–17.

■ SEE QUESTIONS: 33, 88, 148

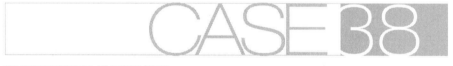

WATERSHED INFARCTS

OBJECTIVES

▨ To review the clinical characteristics of watershed infarctions.
▨ To discuss the pathogenetic mechanisms of watershed infarctions.

VIGNETTE

A 65-year-old woman with a T4, N1, M0 squamous cell carcinoma of the left retromalar trigone and mandible had a composite resection with modified radical neck dissection and tracheostomy followed by a free flap reconstruction. On the morning after surgery, the patient appeared slightly less responsive and remained ventilated. Eventually the patient became more responsive. However, she continued to have poor movements of all her extremities.

CASE SUMMARY

Our patient had a perioperative stroke. Cerebral hemodynamics seems to be a very important factor in the production of a perioperative stroke. Symptomatic patients with severe carotid artery disease may be at high risk of perioperative watershed infarction.

The watershed cortical areas are the first to be deprived of sufficient blood flow in the event of cerebral hypoperfusion. Watershed infarcts occur in the border zone between adjacent arterial perfusion beds. The mechanism whereby watershed infarcts occur remains controversial. Although most authors suggest that watershed infarctions arise from hemodynamic derangements, cerebral embolization may also be a common cause, as there is evidence for a preferential distribution of emboli to the cerebral arterial borderzone regions.

During or after cardiac surgery or after an episode of sustained and severe arterial hypotension after cardiac arrest, prolonged hypoxemia, or bilateral severe carotid artery disease (as in our patient), ischemia may occur in the watershed areas between the major circulations. Watershed infarcts also may be unilateral when there is some degree of hemodynamic failure in patients with underlying severe arterial stenosis or occlusion and a noncompetent circle of Willis. Watershed infarcts also may be caused by microembolic processes or hyperviscosity states and have been reported after near-drowning events.

Ischemia in the border-zone territory of the anterior cerebral artery (ACA), middle cerebral artery (MCA), and posterior cerebral artery (PCA) may result in bilateral parietooccipital infarcts. There can be a variety of visual manifestations, including bilateral lower altitudinal field defects, optic ataxia, cortical blindness, and difficulty in judging size, distance, and movement. Ischemia between the territories of the ACA and MCA bilaterally may result in bibrachial cortical sensorimotor impairment (man in a barrel) and impaired saccadic eye movements caused by compromise of the frontal eye fields.

Ischemia on the border-zone regions between the MCA and PCA may cause bilateral parietotemporal infarctions. Initially, there is cortical blindness that may improve, but defects such as dyslexia, dyscalculia, dysgraphia, and memory defects for verbal and nonverbal material may persist. Watershed infarcts are also recognized between the territorial supply of the posterior inferior cerebellar artery (PICA), anterior inferior cerebellar artery (AICA), and superior cerebellar artery (SCA). Watershed infarcts may also involve the internal watershed region of the centrum semiovale alongside and slightly above the body of the lateral ventricles, and in the spinal cord.

■ SELECTED REFERENCES

Biller J, ed. *Practical neurology,* 2nd ed. Philadelphia: Lippincott Williams & Wilkins, 2002.

Brazis PW, Masdeu JC, Biller J. *Localization in clinical neurology,* 4th ed. Philadelphia: Lippincott Williams & Wilkins, 2001.

Gerraty RP, Gilford EJ, Gates PC. Watershed cerebral infarction associated with perioperative hypotension. *Clin Exp Neurol* 1993;30:82–89.

Graeber MC, Jordan JE, Mishra SK, et al. Watershed infarction on computed tomographic scan. An unreliable sign of hemodynamic stroke. *Arch Neurol* 1992;49:311–313.

■ SEE QUESTIONS: 20, 116, 117, 118, 119, 120, 121, 122, 123, 138, 139, 179

CASE 39

MOYAMOYA SYNDROME ASSOCIATED WITH DOWN SYNDROME

OBJECTIVES

▨ To review the basic pathophysiology of moyamoya disease.
▨ To review the clinical characteristics of moyamoya disease.
▨ To discuss ancillary diagnostic tests in moyamoya disease.
▨ To review management principles in moyamoya disease.

VIGNETTE

At the age of 18, this boy had experienced transient weakness involving the right upper extremity associated with dysarthria and facial weakness.

CASE SUMMARY

Our patient had specific facial features, brachiocephaly, up-slanted and narrow palpebral fissures, shortened digits, hypotonia, and joint hyperextensibility, characteristic of trisomy 21 or Down syndrome. He was also found to have hypothyroidism and sleep apnea, but he had no underlying congenital heart disease. His stroke was felt to be secondary to moyamoya syndrome.

Moyamoya (Japanese for "puff of smoke") disease is a progressive, nonatherosclerotic, noninflammatory, occlusive disease of the cerebral vasculature of unknown etiology with particular involvement of the terminal portions of the internal carotid arteries and the circle of Willis. It is characterized by stenosis or occlusion of the distal intracranial internal carotid artery or the adjacent anterior, middle, or posterior cerebral arteries, along with the development of stereotypical collaterals (basal, parenchymal, leptomeningeal, or dural). Moyamoya disease, seen in both children and young adults, has a bimodal age distribution with a peak in the first and fourth decades of life. Half of the affected patients present before 10 years of age and familial occurrence has been reported. Pathologically, there is fibrocellular thickening of the intima, waving of the internal elastic lamina, and attenuation of the media.

Proposed criteria for the diagnosis of moyamoya disease are stenosis or occlusion involving the region of the internal carotid artery bifurcation (C1) and proximal portions of the anterior cerebral artery (A1) and middle cerebral arteries (M1), presence of unusual netlike (puff of smoke) appearance of basal collateral arteries arising from the circle of Willis, and bilateral abnormalities. Occasionally, these abnormalities are found in association with a variety of other disease states, and the angiographic abnormality in those instances is called moyamoya syndrome rather than moyamoya disease.

Many disease states have been associated with moyamoya. These include neonatal anoxia, trauma, basilar meningitis, tuberculous meningitis, leptospirosis, cranial irradiation therapy for optic pathway gliomas, neurofibromatosis type 1 (von Recklinghausen disease), tuberous sclerosis, brain tumors, fibromuscular dysplasia, polyarteritis nodosa, Marfan syndrome, pseudoxanthoma elasticum, hypomelanosis of Ito, Williams syndrome, Turner syndrome, Alagille syndrome, cerebral dissecting and saccular aneurysms, sickle cell anemia, β thalassemia, aplastic anemia, Fanconi anemia, Apert syndrome, factor XII deficiency, type I glycogenosis, NADH-coenzyme Q reductase deficiency, renal artery stenosis, coarctation of the aorta, and Down syndrome.

Clinical presentation in young adults with moyamoya disease can include hemiparesis, monoparesis, alternating hemiparesis, early morning headaches and nausea, seizures, involuntary (mostly choreiform) movements, intellectual decline, mental retardation, cerebral infarction, and intracranial hemorrhage. In adults, the most common symptoms are hemorrhagic, caused by subarachnoid, subependymal, or intraventricular hemorrhage. Ischemic strokes may be multiple and recurrent and predominantly involve the carotid circulation. The infarctions may be superficial or deep and often involve watershed territories.

Routine hematological, biochemical, and serologic investigations are unrevealing except for reports of elevated fibroblastic growth factor in the cerebrospinal fluid. Cerebral angiography is the gold standard for diagnosis. The diagnosis is based on a distinct arteriographic appearance characterized by bilateral stenosis or occlusion of the terminal portion of the internal carotid arteries with frequent involvement of the circle of Willis and development of an extensive collateral vascular network at the base of the brain in the vicinity of the stenotic or occlusive areas. MRA may preclude the need for conventional angiography if surgery is not anticipated.

The optimal treatment for moyamoya disease has not yet been determined. Platelet antiaggregants, calcium channel blockers, corticosteroids, vasodilators, and antifibrinolytics have been used. Surgical revascularization has been used in the management of the ischemic complications of childhood moyamoya. Various surgical procedures have been used. These procedures are divided into two groups depending on whether they involve direct or indirect anastomosis. Revascularization surgery is less useful in patients presenting with intracranial hemorrhage.

■ SELECTED REFERENCES

Hoffman H. Moyamoya disease and syndrome. *Clin Neurol Neurosurg* 1997;99:S39–S44.
Pearson E, Lenn NJ, Cail WS. Moyamoya and other causes of stroke in patients with Down syndrome. *Pediatr Neurol* 1985;1(May-Jun):174–179.

■ SEE QUESTIONS: 29, 30, 46, 78, 141, 203

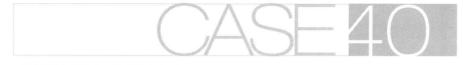

TAKAYASU'S ARTERITIS

OBJECTIVES

- To review the basic pathophysiology of the vasculitides.
- To review the clinical characteristics of Takayasu's arteritis.
- To discuss ancillary diagnostic tests in Takayasu's arteritis.
- To review management principles in Takayasu's arteritis.

VIGNETTE

A 36-year-old woman had a history of erythema nodosum (for which she received prednisone) and generalized fatigue and achiness in both shoulders, hips, and back. For the last 3 years, she had felt very tired and described her symptoms as like having the flu all the time.

The patient was seen by numerous physicians and apparently a conclusive diagnosis was never reached. She was also found to be anemic and further investigations were undertaken to evaluate her gastrointestinal (GI) tract. In addition, she had a history of uveitis of the left eye and bilateral episcleritis.

More recently, she developed achiness around her neck, particularly on the right side, left arm pain and weakness with effort, and episodes of visual "whiteouts" when exposed to bright light. Her blood pressure (BP) was 140/90 mm Hg on the right arm and not obtainable on the left arm. The left radial pulse was not palpable. There were harsh right-sided cervical bruits.

CASE SUMMARY

Vascular injury is the central pathology in the vasculitides and the mechanisms of injury are diverse. Vasculitis is characterized by blood vessel inflammation and necrosis.

Four basic types of immunopathogenetic mechanisms have been accepted: I, anaphylactic type; II, cytotoxic/cell activating type; III, immune complex type; and IV, cell-mediated type. Injury can also occur by other pathways including direct cytokine mediated, direct neutrophil involvement, genetically mediated, direct infectious, or environmental/chemical injury. More than one mechanism is likely to be involved in a particular vasculitis. The diagnosis of vasculitis is often inferential, based on clinical presentation, presence of multisystem organ involvement, and abnormal serologic tests.

Takayasu's arteritis (TA) is a chronic panarteritis localized to the aortic arch or its branches, the ascending thoracic aorta, the abdominal aorta, or the entire aorta. TA, also known as pulseless disease, is more common in women than in men. TA has two distinctive phases: a prepulseless (inflammatory or systemic) phase and a pulseless phase. Systemic symptoms of TA include fatigue, weight loss, low-grade fever, arthralgias, thoracic back pain, and new-onset hypertension. Other systemic related symptoms include vertigo when looking upward, syncope, convulsions, dementia, claudication in one arm or leg, ischemia of the extremities, ischemic optic neuropathy, and decreased visual acuity. Widespread bruits, a weak or absent radial pulse, and differences in blood pressure between both arms are helpful diagnostic clues. Intermittent claudication of jaw muscles and atrophy of the facial musculature may be evident.

Diagnosis of TA is confirmed by aortic angiography or 3D CT angiography. MRI and MRA are valuable noninvasive diagnostic tools. Laboratory abnormalities may include anemia, leukocytosis, increased erythrocyte sedimentation rate (ESR), elevated C-reactive protein (CRP), and hypergammaglobulinemia.

Management includes glucocorticoids. Antiplatelet therapy is often used to prevent thrombus formation. Surgical reconstructive methods or percutaneous transluminal angioplasty are often needed for the chronic arterial lesions of TA.

■ **SELECTED REFERENCES**

Fraga A, Mint G, Valle L, et al. Takayasu's arteritis: frequency of systemic manifestations (study of 22 patients) and favorable response to maintenance steroid therapy with adrenocorticosteroids (12 patients). *Arthritis Rheum* 1977;15:617–624.

Lupi-Herrera E, Sanchez-Torres G, Marcushamer J, et al. Takayasu's arteritis. Clinical study of 107 cases. *Am Heart J* 1977;93:94–103.

■ **SEE QUESTIONS: 29, 45, 94**

CASE 41

RECURRENT FACIAL PALSIES (VZV) FOLLOWED BY CEREBRAL INFARCTION

OBJECTIVES

■ To review the clinical characteristics of Ramsay-Hunt syndrome (herpes zoster oticus).
■ To analyze the different vasculopathies associated with varicella-zoster virus (VZV) infection.

VIGNETTE

A 47-year-old left-handed man had chickenpox at approximately 7 years of age. For as long as he can remember after that, he had intermittent right-hand painful blisters as well as painful blisters on the right side of the posterior neck at the hairline associated with unilateral headaches.

In July 1997, at age 41, he had a cerebral infarction and was found to have an occluded right internal carotid artery and 9% stenosis of the left internal carotid artery. He had a left carotid endarterectomy.

His clinical course was unremarkable until September 1998 when he developed a right peripheral facial weakness associated with vesicles on his right ear. Over the past 4 years, he has had at least two to three episodes per year of the vesicular rash on the palm of the right hand and posterior neck at the hairline, each time associated with severe right-sided headaches and a recurrent left peripheral facial paralysis a few years after his stroke.

CASE SUMMARY

Our patient had acute facial paralysis associated with herpetic vesicles of the skin of the external auditory canal, suggesting that he had Ramsay-Hunt syndrome, also known as herpes zoster oticus, geniculate neuralgia, or nervus intermedius neuralgia. The vesicles may also appear on the pinna, tympanic membrane, or in the soft palate and anterior two-thirds of the tongue. Subsequently, our patient developed a hemispheric cerebral infarction probably associated with varicella-zoster virus (VZV) infection. Besides acute facial paralysis and intense otalgia on the affected side, patients with Ramsay-Hunt syndrome may also have vertigo, ipsilateral tinnitus, and ipsilateral hearing loss. Unlike patients with Bell"s palsy, patients with Ramsay-Hunt syndrome have a complete recovery of less than 50%.

VZV causes chickenpox (varicella) and shingles (herpes zoster). VZV is associated with large or small vessel vasculopathy and may also cause a virus-induced necrotizing arteritis similar to granulomatous angiitis of the CNS. CNS large vessel vasculitis developing between 4 to 6 weeks after herpes zoster ophthalmicus is the most common VZV vasculitis. Cerebral angiography often demonstrates unilateral segmental narrowing of the proximal segments of the middle, anterior, or, less common, the posterior cerebral or internal carotid artery. CSF may show a discrete lymphocytic pleocytosis. Intravenous acyclovir is the treatment of choice for complicated VZV infections. Other options include valacyclovir, famciclovir, or ganciclovir. Uncommonly, a postvaricella angiopathy affecting small and large vessels may develop. Pathologic studies have demonstrated changes consistent with vasculitis with lymphocytic infiltration of the vessel walls.

■ SELECTED REFERENCES

Hilt DC, Buchholz D, Krumholz A, et al. Herpes zoster ophthalmicus and delayed contralateral hemiparesis caused by cerebral angiitis: diagnosis and management approaches. *Ann Neurol* 1983;14:543–553.
Robillard RB, Hilsinger RL, Adour KK. Ramsay Hunt facial paralysis: clinical analyses of 185 patients. *Otolaryngol Head Neck Surg* 1986;95:292–297.

■ SEE QUESTIONS: 83, 87, 148, 152, 157, 158, 164, 165

CASE 42

MULTIPLE LOBAR HEMORRHAGES DUE TO CEREBRAL AMYLOID ANGIOPATHY

OBJECTIVES

- ▦ To review the clinical characteristics of lobar intracerebral hemorrhages.
- ▦ To discuss nonhypertensive causes of intracerebral hemorrhages.
- ▦ To illustrate a unique form of cerebral angiopathy.

VIGNETTE

A 56-year-old normotensive man consulted us because of recurrent lobar intracerebral hemorrhages.

CASE SUMMARY

Our nonhypertensive patient had multiple bilateral recurrent lobar posterior intracerebral hemorrhages over a period of months. *Intracranial hemorrhage* is defined as any bleed occurring within the cranial cavity. Intracranial hemorrhage may be located in the epidural, subdural, subarachnoid, parenchymal, or intraventricular compartment. Intracerebral hemorrhage accounts for 10% to 15% of all strokes. The most common causes of nontraumatic intracerebral hemorrhage in adults are those related to arterial hypertension (50% to 70% of cases). Hypertensive hemorrhages tend to occur in specific sites (putamen, thalamus, subcortical white matter, cerebellum, and pons).

Intracerebral hemorrhage may present clinically in very much the same way as an ischemic stroke. The presence of severe arterial hypertension or a bleeding diathesis, as well as headache and vomiting, favors a diagnosis of intracerebral hemorrhage. There are general features of the clinical syndrome of intracerebral hemorrhage that may help to characterize it. Historical features include a presentation that is maximum at the onset in one-third of patients and gradual with smooth progression over 30 minutes in two-thirds of patients.

Most hemorrhages occur during activity rather than during sleep. A headache is present in approximately one-half of patients. Nausea and vomiting are present in over 50% of patients. The level of consciousness may be variable. Seizures rarely occur at the onset. There is usually no history of any prodromal attack. There is often a history of arterial hypertension. On examination, meningeal irritation signs can be seen if the bleeding extends to the subarachnoid space. Retinal hemorrhages may be present on funduscopic examination.

The various forms of intracerebral hemorrhages have distinctive clinical presentations that are dependent on the location, size, direction of spread, and the rate of development of the bleeding. A lobar intracerebral hemorrhage refers to bleeding occurring within the subcortical supratentorial white matter located outside the deep nuclear structures. About 23% of lobar intracerebral hemorrhages occur in the subcortical white matter. Underlying structural lesions are more common than arterial hypertension as a cause. The clinical presentation can resemble that of an embolic cerebral infarction.

Lobar intracerebral hemorrhages may be due to a specific etiologic factor. Lobar intracerebral hemorrhages can arise from a wide variety of origins including ruptured cerebral arteriovenous and cavernous malformations, ruptured intracranial aneurysms, bleeding diatheses, primary or metastatic tumors, cerebral venous occlusive disease, oral anticoagulant use, thrombolytic therapy, sympathomimetic drug use (cocaine, amphetamines, phenylpropanolamine), arterial hypertension, vasculitis, infectious disorders, following surgical procedures, or cerebral amyloid angiopathy.

Frontal hemorrhages may result in contralateral hemiparesis and abulia. Conjugate deviation of the eyes toward the side of the hematoma may occur. Bifrontal headache is frequently reported. Parietal lobe hemorrhages may cause contralateral hemisensory loss and neglect of the contralateral visual field. These hematomas may also cause variable degrees of contralateral homonymous hemianopia, mild hemiparesis, and anosognosia. Dominant temporal lobe hemorrhages may cause Wernicke's aphasia. Hematomas affecting the left temporoparietal area can also result in conduction or global aphasia. Temporal lobe hemorrhages may also cause visual field defects, headaches around or anterior to the ipsilateral ear, and occasionally, a syndrome of agitated delirium. Occipital lobe hemorrhages are characterized by ipsilateral orbital pain and contralateral homonymous hemianopia.

Because many conditions may cause intracerebral hemorrhage, patients suspected of it deserved a thorough evaluation. Unenhanced CT is still the safest, most effective method currently available to identify accurately the location, site, direction of extension, and type of acute intracerebral hemorrhage. MRI is an important tool for identifying bleeding lesions such as vascular malformations and/or tumors. Gradient echo MRI techniques are extremely useful in detecting small petechial hemorrhages or areas of hemosiderin deposition. Catheter cerebral angiography is of importance when there is reason to suspect an aneurysm, arteriovenous malformation, vasculitis, or moyamoya disease. Cerebral angiography is also often performed in patients who have an atypical location for hypertensive hemorrhage or in the young patient who is not hypertensive.

After extensive investigations excluded the most common causes of recurrent lobar intracerebral hemorrhage, based on cortical involvement, multiplicity, bilaterality, and the recurrent nature of the intracerebral hemorrhages in our patient, we believe that he most likely had cerebral amyloid angiopathy (CAA, congophilic angiopathy). Hemorrhages secondary to CAA are usually large and multiple. As in our patient, there is a predilection for the parietaloccipital regions.

CAA is characterized by amyloid deposition in the leptomeningeal, cortical, and subcortical medium- and small-sized arteries and arterioles. Pathologically, amyloid is stained pink with Congo red and shows a characteristic yellow-green birefringence under polarized light. Different biochemical types of amyloid have been identified. The amyloid peptide (A4), a cleavage product of amyloid precursor protein, is usually found in patients with Alzheimer disease, Down syndrome, or in older but otherwise healthy individuals.

CAA is also encountered in the Dutch variant of hereditary cerebral hemorrhage with amyloid angiopathy (HCDWA-D), in the Icelandic type of hereditary cerebral hemorrhage with amyloidosis, and in a rare variant associated with nonneuritic plaques and dementia. The Icelandic type is related to a mutation of the cystalin C gene. CAA is also associated with dementia pugilistica, Creutzfeldt-Jakob disease, cerebellar ataxia, granulomatous angiitis, rheumatoid vasculitis, giant cell arteritis, postradiation necrosis, and vascular malformations. CAA is associated with apolipoprotein epsilon, E-epsilon 4 (APDE-epsilon 4) allele. The APDE-epsilon 4 allele is associated with an earlier onset of intracerebral hemorrhage in CAA.

Severe CAA can cause lobar intracerebral hemorrhage, dementia with leukoencephalopathy, and transient neurological deficits. CAA is the most common cause of lobar hemorrhages in older normotensive individuals. It has been estimated that approximately 20% of patients with CAA eventually have intracerebral bleeding. CAA-associated hemorrhages are often located close to the cortical surface and often rupture into the subarachnoid space. Cerebellum or pontine involvement is exceptional. Subdural hematomas and subarachnoid hemorrhage can occur. It is likely that CAA may play a role in some cases of intracerebral hemorrhage associated with the administration of tPA.

Treatment of intracerebral hemorrhage due to CAA is controversial. No medical therapy is available. Platelet antiaggregants or nonsteroidal antiinflammatory drugs should be avoided. Surgery can be performed for symptomatic treatment.

■ **SELECTED REFERENCES**

Greenberg SM. Genetics of primary intracerebral hemorrhage. *Semin Cerebrovasc Dis Stroke* 2002;2:59–65.
Izumihara A, Ishihara T, Iwamoto N, et al. Postoperative outcome of 37 patients with lobar intracerebral hemorrhage related to cerebral amyloid angiopathy. *Stroke* 1999;30:29–33.
Kase CS, Williams JP, Wyatt DA, et al. Lobar intracerebral hematomas: clinical and CT analysis of 22 cases. *Neurology* 1982;32:1146.
Pendlebury WW, Iole ED, Tracy RP, et al. Intracerebral hemorrhage related to cerebral amyloid angiopathy and tPA. *Ann Neurol* 1991;29:210–213.

■ **SEE QUESTIONS: 52, 66, 71, 93, 104, 178, 188, 216, 217, 220, 221, 223**

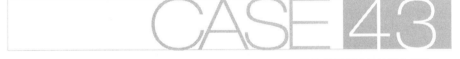

PURE SENSORY STROKE DUE TO THALAMIC HEMORRHAGE

OBJECTIVES

- To describe the clinical characteristics of pure sensory stroke (pure hemisensory or paresthetic stroke).
- To highlight the fact that discrete hemorrhages can account for this and other lacunar syndromes.

VIGNETTE

A 61-year-old African-American woman with a history of poorly controlled hypertension was evaluated because of the acute onset of left hemibody numbness. Her BP was 204/100 mm Hg.

CASE SUMMARY

Acute stroke is one of the leading causes of morbidity and mortality in the world. It is estimated to be the third leading cause of death in the United States. Stroke is a clinical diagnosis that requires a prompt diagnostic evaluation in the emergency room. Differentiation between infarction and hemorrhage is paramount. In the Western world, 80% to 85% of strokes are ischemic; the rest are hemorrhagic. Hemorrhagic strokes are defined as either intraparenchymal or subarachnoid and occur in about 15% to 20% of acute strokes. Thoroughness with the history and physical examination is essential in guiding a rational and cost-effective paraclinical evaluation.

Our patient had uncontrolled arterial hypertension and presented to the emergency room fully alert and with a pure sensory stroke. Physicians in the emergency room initially interpreted her deficits as the result of a subcortical ischemic lesion. However, the CT scan showed a small hypertensive thalamic hemorrhage. Hypertension is the most important modifiable risk factor for coronary heart disease, stroke, congestive heart failure, end-stage renal disease, and peripheral vascular disease.

Pure sensory stroke (pure hemisensory or paresthetic stroke) is characterized by unilateral numbness, paresthesias, and a hemisensory deficit involving the face, arm, trunk, and leg. Subjective complaints may be out of proportion to objective findings. Lacunae in the ventroposterolateral nucleus of the thalamus may cause this syndrome. Pure sensory stroke can also be due to ischemic infarctions in the corona radiata or in the parietal cortex.

Pure sensory stroke, also known as pure paresthetic stroke or pure hemisensory stroke, is often due to a lacune involving the ventroposterolateral nucleus of the thalamus. It is characterized by numbness, paresthesias, and a unilateral hemisensory deficit involving the face, arm, trunk, and leg. Subjective symptoms often predominate over objective findings in this syndrome. Sensory symptoms due to stroke often produce distal manifestations in the form of cheirooral, cheiropedal, or cheirooral-pedal syndromes. Only rarely, the sensory manifestations are restricted to proximal body segments. Small ischemic strokes in the internal capsule/corona radiata, subthalamus, midbrain, or in the parietal cortex may also cause a pure sensory stroke, as may pontine lacunes localized in the medial lemniscus or paramedian dorsal pons.

Differentiation of a pontine pure sensory syndrome from a thalamic pure sensory syndrome may be difficult. Brainstem pure sensory strokes often show a discrepancy between superficial and deep sensations. In pontine pure sensory stroke, vibration and position sense are often reduced on the paresthetic side, whereas sensation to pinprick and temperature are preserved. Conversely, in cases of pure sensory stroke involving the thalamus, internal capsule, or corona radiata, both spinothalamic and medial lemniscal modalities are compromised. Likewise, ipsilateral impairment of smooth pursuit and vestibuloocular reflex may indicate a pontine lesion in patients with hemisensory stroke. A pure sensory deficit affecting pain and temperature sensation may also be due to a small hemorrhage in the dorsolateral midbrain.

In a report of 21 patients with pure sensory stroke, 11 patients had thalamic strokes, 7 patients had lacunes or hemorrhages in the leticulocapsular region or corona radiata, 2 had pontine tegmental strokes, and 1 had a small cortical infarct. Hemisensory deficits of all modalities usually were associated with a relatively large lacune or hemorrhage in the lateral thalamus, whereas tract-specific or restricted sensory changes suggested very small strokes in the sensory pathway from the pons to the parietal cortex.

■ SELECTED REFERENCES

Biller J, ed. *Practical neurology*, 2nd ed. Philadelphia: Lippincott Williams & Wilkins, 2002.

Brazis PW, Masdeu JC, Biller J. *Localization in clinical neurology*, 4th ed. Philadelphia: Lippincott Williams & Wilkins, 2001.

■ SEE QUESTIONS: 35, 39, 47, 55, 71, 93, 104, 188, 216, 217, 233

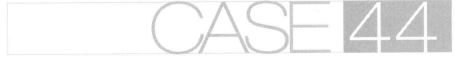

SUPERIOR SAGITTAL SINUS THROMBOSIS

OBJECTIVES

- To discuss the clinical presentation of cerebral venous thrombosis.
- To discuss the management of sagittal sinus thrombosis.
- To discuss the management of anticoagulant therapy in pregnancy.

VIGNETTE

A 30-year-old woman was seen 3 years ago because of severe frontal headaches. After 3 days of headaches and dizziness, she noted that her left leg was "limp." Then her left arm became weak, and she also had slurred speech and left facial weakness. Subsequently, she had a spell characterized by turning of her head to the left and jerking of her left extremities with secondary generalization. She was diagnosed as having a superior sagittal sinus thrombosis. The only abnormality found was an increased IgA antiphosphatidylethanolamine antibody. She was treated with heparin and was discharged on warfarin. More than 1 year later, she became pregnant.

CASE SUMMARY

At the age of 27, our patient suddenly experienced a severe right frontal headache associated with left leg weakness. Cranial computed tomography (CT) showed a small right frontal hemorrhage. Magnetic resonance imaging (MRI) showed a hemorrhagic infarction involving the right frontoparietal lobe and the left posterior parietal lobe. Magnetic resonance venography (MRV) and catheter cerebral angiography (venous phase) documented an occlusion of the anterior portion of the superior sagittal sinus. Subsequently, the patient had a single seizure characterized by head deviation to the left, followed by rhythmic clonic movements of the left arm and leg, followed by loss of consciousness. She received intravenous phenytoin and was referred for further evaluation and management.

Her past medical history was fairly unremarkable except for abruptio placenta at 8 months gestation. She smoked a pack of cigarettes daily and was not on oral contraceptives. General physical examination showed extensive livedo reticularis. There was residual weakness of her left hamstrings, foot dorsiflexors, and plantar flexors. Patellar and Achilles reflexes were brisk (left greater than right). Ancillary investigations showed persistent elevation of IgA antiphosphatidylethanolamine titers. She was treated with intravenous unfractionated heparin followed by warfarin. She also received oral phenytoin and folic acid.

Three years later, while still on warfarin, she became pregnant. She stopped warfarin on the first day she recognized she was late for her menses. Neurologic reexamination was stable. A fetal ultrasound was normal.

The patient was treated with 81 mg of aspirin daily and subcutaneous enoxaparin (initially 60 mg bid and then 80 mg bid). She also received folic acid, prenatal vitamins, vitamin D, and calcium supplements. On her thirty-seventh week of gestation, the enoxaparin was discontinued and she was started on subcutaneous administration of unfractionated heparin. Following an unremarkable delivery, she was allowed to breastfeed her baby and had been restarted on warfarin.

Intracranial sinovenous occlusive disease is an infrequent cause of stroke although it has a variety of causes. It often causes hemorrhagic infarction. The most common symptoms of cerebral venous thrombosis are headache, seizures, focal neurologic deficits, and altered levels of consciousness. These symptoms may evolve over time. Depending on the vein or sinus involved, the focal signs are typically noted on neurologic examination. A careful fundoscopic examination may reveal bilateral papilledema secondary to an increase in intracranial pressure. The superior sagittal sinus is most frequently involved. Imaging studies often reveal parasagittal lesions. This often leads to lower extremity signs and symptoms.

Head MRI and MR venography often reveal the brain parenchymal abnormalities as well as occlusion of the appropriate larger venous structure. Catheter angiography, typically the venous phase, can also be used to diagnose a cerebral venous thrombosis. It is important to determine whether the venous thrombosis is aseptic or caused by a local infection as the septic thromboses will require appropriate antibiotic treatment. Aseptic intracranial venous thrombosis is divided into dural venous sinus thrombosis, deep venous thrombosis, and superficial or cortical vein thrombosis. A variety of hypercoaguable states have been associated with aseptic venous thrombosis. Antiphospholipid antibodies represent the most common acquired thrombophilic state.

The treatment of an aseptic superior sagittal thrombosis is aimed at the primary underlying pathology and anticoagulants are most commonly used. The most common medications used acutely are unfractionated heparin, low molecular weight heparins, or heparinoids. Warfarin anticoagulation is used longer term. For those with a diagnosed hypercoaguable state, warfarin is used chronically. Anticoagulants are typically used despite the presence of hemorrhagic infarctions. Antiepileptic medications are used for seizure prevention, and appropriate treatment for elevated intracranial pressure is used when necessary. If a patient deteriorates despite anticoagulation, endovascular thrombolysis can be considered. Because warfarin has been associated with an embryopathy, it is not used during pregnancy.

The highest risk of warfarin embryopathy occurs in infants exposed between the sixth and twelfth weeks of gestation. Subcutaneous heparin is often used in pregnant women requiring anticoagulation. There are risks involved in using heparin during pregnancy including osteoporosis, heparin-induced thrombocytopenia (with or without thrombosis), hypoaldosteronism, and alopecia. Calcium and vitamin D should be supplemented because of the risk of osteoporosis. The dose of heparin is often increased in the later stages of pregnancy and may be adjusted by measuring the activated partial thromboplastin time (aPTT). Low molecular weight heparins can be used as a replacement for heparin. Low-dose aspirin (81 mg) may be added to heparin, especially in those with antiphospholipid antibodies. Warfarin may be resumed postpartum.

■ **SELECTED REFERENCES**

Bousser MG, Russel RR. Cerebral venous thrombosis (Monograph). WB Saunders, 1996.

Carhuapoma JR, Mitsias O, Levine SR. Cerebral venous thrombosis and anticardiolipin antibodies. *Neurology* 1997;28:2363–2369.

Kaplan JM, Biller J, Adams HP Jr. Outcome in non-septic spontaneous superior sagittal sinus thrombosis in adults. *Cerebrovasc Dis* 1991;1:231–234.

Rosene-Montella K, Ginsberg J. Thromboembolic disease in pregnancy. In: Elkayam U, Gleicher N, eds. *Cardiac problems in pregnancy.* New York: Wiley-Liss, 1998:223–235.

■ **SEE QUESTIONS: 71, 104, 145, 220, 221, 227**

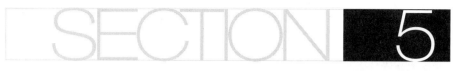

SECTION 5

EXTRAPYRAMIDAL

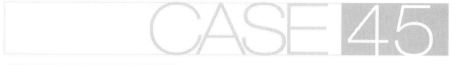

CASE 45

PARKINSONIAN TREMOR

OBJECTIVES

▪ To review the clinical features of parkinsonian tremor.
▪ To illustrate the unusual occurrence of a subcortical infarct that abated the patient's tremor.

VIGNETTE

This 72-year-old woman consulted us because of tremors.

CASE SUMMARY

Our patient had an asymmetric resting tremor (4 to 7 Hz) of her relaxed left hand characteristic of parkinsonian tremor. Tremor consists of rhythmic, oscillating movements of agonist and antagonist muscles. Tremor at rest is seen exclusively in Parkinson's disease and in drug-induced parkinsonism.

The cardinal features of Parkinson's disease are resting tremor, rigidity, bradykinesia, and postural instability. In Parkinson's disease, typical movements include pronation-supination of the forearm and rhythmic movements with alternating opposition of the thumb and fingers (pill-rolling).

The tremor is often markedly asymmetric or purely unilateral at onset. The tremor occurs mainly in the distal part of the limb. Occasionally the tremor reappears when the hands are held in an outstretched posture. A less prominent low-amplitude and higher frequency kinetic tremor is also common. The tremor occasionally also affects the chin, jaw, or tongue. The tremor abates during sleep and worsens with anxiety and stress. This type of tremor almost never involves the head and seldom interferes with activities of daily living.

Following a subcortical infarction in the distribution of the right anterior choroidal artery, not resulting in hemiparesis, our patient's unilateral left hand resting tremor ceased. We hypothesized that this clinical association may be similar to the pioneering observations of Dr. Irving Cooper, who treated some patients with tremor by creating deep lesions with either anterior choroidal artery ligation or cryogenic thalamotomy.

■ SELECTED REFERENCES

Biller J, ed. *Practical neurology,* 2nd ed. Philadelphia: Lippincott Williams & Wilkins, 2002.

Brazis PW, Masdeu JC, Biller J. *Localization in clinical neurology,* 4th ed. Philadelphia: Lippincott Williams & Wilkins, 2001.

Rosenow J, Das K, Rovit RL, et al. Irving S. Cooper and his role in intracranial stimulation for movement disorders and epilepsy. *Stereotactic Funct Neurosurg* 2002;78:95–112.

■ SEE QUESTIONS: 40, 41, 42, 52, 60, 107, 125, 126, 169, 170, 234

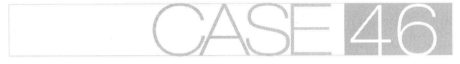

CASE 46

ESSENTIAL TREMOR

OBJECTIVES

▨ To review the clinical features of essential tremor.
▨ To discuss the differential diagnosis of essential tremor.
▨ To summarize medical and surgical management options for essential tremor.

VIGNETTE

This 75-year-old woman was evaluated because of hand tremors.

CASE SUMMARY

Our patient had tremor of her hands, head, and voice. The tremor interfered with her handwriting and drawing and affected her social life. The tremor was not present at rest. She had some suppression of the tremor from the ingestion of small amounts of alcohol. There were no other neurologic symptoms or signs. There was no family history of tremor.

Tremor consists of rhythmic, oscillating movements of agonist and antagonist muscles. Our patient had characteristic features for essential tremor. Essential tremor, the most common hyperkinetic movement disorder, is characterized by a slowly progressive postural and/or kinetic tremor, usually affecting both hands and forearms and less commonly the head and voice. Involvement of the face, trunk, and lower limbs is rare. This disorder affects men and women equally. Age of onset has been reported to be bimodal with peaks in the second and sixth decades or unimodal, peaking in the fifth decade. Most frequently, the tremor affects the hands followed by the head and voice. The tremor usually begins in one upper extremity and soon compromises the other. A mild degree of asymmetry is not uncommon.

Essential tremor usually presents with flexion and extension movements of the upper limbs with a frequency of 5 to 10 Hz. The tremor frequency decreases with advanced age. The tremor is characteristically absent at rest, present with maintained posture, and most evident at the end of a goal-directed movement. Essential tremor rarely affects the jaw. Essential tremor may be sporadic or hereditary. Essential tremor is familial in 50% to 70% of cases, with most patients inheriting the disorder through an autosomal dominant gene. An association with dystonia and Parkinson's disease has been reported. Hyperthyroidism, and drugs such as lithium and valproic acid can exacerbate an underlying essential tremor. Differential diagnostic considerations most often include Parkinson's disease and dystonic tremor.

Management with primidone and propranolol are the first line of therapy for essential tremor. Propranolol is usually favored for younger patients and primidone for older individuals. Many other medications have been reported to be of benefit in the management of essential tremor including gabapentin, topiramate, benzodiazepines, clonidine, clozapine, olanzapine, flunarizine, carbonic anhydrase inhibitors, and theophylline. The use of botulinum toxin may be of value for some patients. Surgical treatment for essential tremor has been used for decades. For patients with medically refractory and disabling upper extremity tremor, stereotactic thalamotomy and thalamic stimulation are the procedures of choice. The optimal target is the ventralis intermedius (VIM) nucleus of the thalamus. Thalamotomy has been reported to improve contralateral tremor in 90% of patients.

■ SELECTED REFERENCES

Biller J, ed. *Practical neurology,* 2nd ed. Philadelphia: Lippincott Williams & Wilkins, 2002.

Elble RJ. Diagnostic criteria for essential tremor and differential diagnosis. *Neurology* 2000;11[Suppl 4]: S2–S6.

Koller WC, Hristova A, Brin M. Pharmacologic treatment of essential tremor. *Neurology* 2000;11[Suppl 4]: S30–S38.

Pahwa R, Lyons K, Koller WC. Surgical treatment of essential tremor. *Neurology* 2000;11[Suppl 4]:S39–S44.

■ SEE QUESTIONS: 60, 107, 125, 126, 169, 234

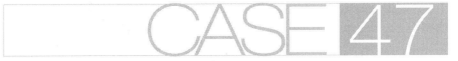

PARKINSONIAN PLUS ESSENTIAL TREMOR

OBJECTIVE

▨ To review the clinical features of a patient with a mixed type of tremor.

VIGNETTE

A 69-year-old man was evaluated because of hand tremors.

CASE SUMMARY

Our patient had an asymmetric tremor of his hands (left greater than right) that interfered with his handwriting, which became micrographic. He also had difficulty using his hands for fine dexterous activities. The tremor worsened with anxiety and stress and abated during sleep. The tremor did not involve his forearms, wrists, head, voice, chin, lips, or tongue. There was no spread of the tremor to his lower extremities, and there was no suppression of the tremor from the ingestion of alcohol. There was a very mild tremor at rest.

A discrete coarse static tremor was also present when the hands were outstretched and was more evident with the usage of the limb at the end of a goal-directed movement. The speech was slightly softer. He also had some degree of facial bradykinesia, mild cogwheeling rigidity on the left wrist detected when the patient drew imaginary circles with his right hand (not shown on the tape), and slight asymmetric reduction of arm swing (left greater than right). He did not have postural instability on the pull test. There was no family history of tremor or Parkinson's disease.

Our patient was diagnosed as having a mixed (parkinsonian and essential tremor) tremor. As many as 20% of patients with Parkinson's disease (PD) have a superimposed essential tremor. The associated postural tremor may precede the onset of PD symptoms for several years. In patients with Parkinson's disease, the degree of rigidity does not correlate with the degree of tremor or bradykinesia. Essential tremor has been associated with Parkinson's disease, dystonia, and certain inherited peripheral neuropathies.

■ SELECTED REFERENCES

Elble RJ. Diagnostic criteria for essential tremor and differential diagnosis. *Neurology* 2000;11[Suppl 4]: S2–S6.

Evidente VG. Understanding essential tremor. Differential diagnosis and options for treatment. *Postgrad Med* 2000;108(Oct):138–140, 143–146, 149.

■ SEE QUESTIONS: 40, 41, 42, 60, 107, 125, 126, 169, 170, 234

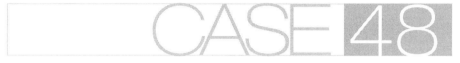

PARKINSON'S DISEASE

OBJECTIVES

▨ To review the clinical features of Parkinson's disease.
▨ To list the differential diagnosis of parkinsonism.
▨ To summarize treatment options for Parkinson's disease.

VIGNETTE

A 56-year-old man had a progressive history of right-sided weakness, lack of dexterity, slowness, and trouble with writing. He also noted a different character of his voice and frequently has had trouble speaking. On occasions, he has had difficulty swallowing medications but no trouble while eating. He has noted some urinary urgency, a weak stream, and mild nocturia. He has had no cognitive problems.

CASE SUMMARY

Our patient is a 56-year-old man who presented with a 3- to 4-year history of slowly progressive decline in function of the right arm and leg. Initially he had difficulty using the gas and brake pedals while driving, and subsequently, difficulty from slowing of arm activities such as brushing his teeth, combing hair, buttoning clothes, and other activities of daily living. While walking he would drag the right foot and hold his right arm in an elevated position.

Neurological examination demonstrates bradykinesia with hypomimia (masked facies), decreased blink frequency, and hypophonia with soft mumbling and monotonous speech. There is an overall paucity of spontaneous movements and decreased amplitude of movements. Handwriting is small (micrographia) and effortful. No tremor is present at rest or with the arms outstretched. There is asymmetric oscillating cogwheel rigidity (right greater than left) detected by passive movements of the limbs. His gait shows short stride and reduced arm swing (right greater than left) and there is mild postural instability.

The four cardinal features of Parkinson's disease are as follows:

1. Resting tremor (although the tremor may be present to some degree while maintaining a posture or with movement of the limbs)
2. Cogwheel rigidity (best established with testing passive resistance at the wrist)
3. Bradykinesia (including masked facies, decreased blink frequency, paucity of spontaneous movements, slow responses, low pitched mumbling voice)
4. Impairment of postural reflexes (poor balance)

Additionally, the diagnosis is often suspected based on simply observing the patient while walking as the steps tend to be short and at times shuffling, associated with a somewhat bent over posture (simian posture) and reduced arm swing (reduced arm synkinesis). Small handwriting (micrographia) is another common feature. Overall, the symptoms and signs tend to be asymmetric and progress over decades. In general, laboratory studies are unhelpful in trying to establish the diagnosis, other than ruling out other conditions that might mimic Parkinson's disease. Nearly all patients with PD respond to dopaminergic therapy.

The differential diagnosis of Parkinsonism is extensive. It is mandatory to look at the patient's medication list to rule out the presence of dopamine blockers. Patients receiving neuroleptics for psychiatric disease, those receiving antiemetics such as prochlorperazine (Compazine), and those receiving metoclopramide (Reglan) should have their medications reviewed and adjusted whenever possible to avoid dopamine blocker exposure. Additionally, patients with recent viral encephalitis, those with exposure to manganese, carbon monoxide poisoning, and some with normal pressure hydrocephalus can demonstrate degrees of parkinsonism. A variety of progressive degenerative brain diseases are associated with variable degrees of parkinsonism.

Progressive supranuclear palsy (PSP) invariably is associated with significant parkinsonism, but the patients have several distinctive features. They have a supranuclear gaze palsy in which initially they have difficulty with volitional downgaze, and as the disease progresses, upgaze and eventually horizontal volitional gaze are affected. Also, in contrast to Parkinson's disease, patients with PSP have more prominent axial or proximal rigidity, less tremor, and a disproportionate degree of speech, swallowing, and balance involvement. Multiple system atrophy presents with parkinsonism in combination with dysautonomia (such as orthostatic hypotension and syncope) in two-thirds of cases, and in one-third of patients multiple system atrophy (MSA) presents with a cerebellar ataxia in association with autonomic insufficiency.

Corticobasal degeneration may also resemble Parkinson's disease. These patients tend to have additional findings including asymmetric or unilateral parietal deficits (alien hand, impaired sensation including astereognosis and agraphesthesia, as well as prominent apraxia and dystonia).

Therapeutic options for Parkinson's disease include a variety of drugs having dopaminergic or anticholinergic effects. Levodopa/carbidopa typically produces striking immediate improvement. In addition, patients with severe depletion of dopaminergic neurons may respond to the addition or substitution of direct dopamine agonists including bromocriptine, pergolide, or pramipexole. Dopaminergic therapy has substantial risks, especially in terms of dyskinesias, including chorea and dystonia, as well as psychiatric side effects of confusion and psychosis. Patients refractory to medical therapy with residual disabling symptoms are candidates for deep brain stimulation.

■ **SELECTED REFERENCES**

Biller J, ed. *Practical neurology,* 2nd ed. Philadelphia: Lippincott Williams & Wilkins, 2002.
Jankovic J. New and emerging therapies for Parkinson's disease. *Arch Neurol* 1999;56:785–790.

Litvan I. Diagnosis and management of progressive supranuclear palsy. *Semin Neurol* 2001;21:41–48.
Tuite P, Ebbitt B. Dopamine agonists. *Semin Neurol* 2001;21:9–14.

■ SEE QUESTIONS: 40, 41, 42, 125, 126, 169, 170

CASE 49

TORTICOLLIS

OBJECTIVES

▓ To illustrate the clinical presentation and diagnosis of cervical dystonia (torticollis).
▓ To outline the common types of focal dystonia.
▓ To summarize the treatment options for disabling focal dystonia.

VIGNETTE

A 58-year-old woman was referred for evaluation of painful spasms of her neck and right shoulder.

CASE SUMMARY

The patient presents with involuntary relatively sustained patterned muscular contractions producing a twisting of the neck and an abnormal posture. Involuntary sustained twisting is referred to as dystonia. Dystonia may be generalized as is the case with acute dystonic reactions from use of dopamine blocking drugs (neuroleptic/antipsychotic medications, antiemetics such as prochlorperazine or metoclopramide for GI symptoms). Generalized dystonia can have a hereditary origin as in dystonia muscularum deformans or be due to cerebral palsy (tension athetoid CP). However, the majority of patients present with a focal or localized dystonia. Focal dystonia commonly affects the cervical muscles, resulting in twisting or pulling of the head to the side commonly referred to as spasmodic torticollis.

Other focal dystonias include blepharospasm (an involuntary closure of the eyelids), dystonic writer's cramp, spasmodic dysphonia, and oromandibular dystonia.

All forms of dystonia tend to be aggravated by stress, anxiety, and fatigue and improve with rest. There may be some degree of fluctuation throughout the day or from week to week, but in general the symptoms are chronic. When patients present with new onset dystonia, it is important to look for recent or concurrent exposure to a dopamine blocking drug (neuroleptic, prochlorperazine, or metoclopramide). Young patients with focal dystonia should be screened for Wilson's disease.

In the majority of patients with focal dystonia, diagnostic testing is relatively normal, making focal dystonia a clinical diagnosis. Ten to 20% of patients may experience spontaneous remission from their focal dystonia, but typically patients will relapse down the road. It is not uncommon for patients to present with chronic neck stiffness or neck pain and undergo an extensive evaluation for disease of the bony spine and disc only to be recognized as having focal dystonia based on clinical observations.

Focal dystonia of the neck may include components of an actual axial twisting referred to as torticollis or tilting to the side (laterocollis), forward flexing (anterocollis), or backward extension (retrocollis). Patients tend to have a stereotyped direction of twisting and posturing and do not alternate from side to side.

Management of focal dystonia, including cervical dystonia, depends on the severity of the patient's symptoms. For mild dystonic phenomenon, no treatment is probably the best approach. On the other hand, for more severe disabling symptoms patients should be considered for a variety of treatment options. The single most effective course of management is botulinum toxin injections, as the vast majority of patients improve usually within a week of the injections and remain so for up to 3 to 6 months, at which point they typically require repeat injection therapy. A long list of medications has been used for treating dystonia over the years and occasionally patients will have a gratifying response to either anticholinergic drugs or benzodiazepines.

■ SELECTED REFERENCES

Biller J, ed. *Practical neurology,* 2nd ed. Philadelphia: Lippincott Williams & Wilkins, 2002.

Brashear A. The botulinum toxins and the treatment of cervical dystonia. *Semin Neurol* 2001;21:85–90.

■ SEE QUESTIONS: 204, 254, 255

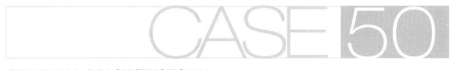

CEREBRAL PALSY/DYSTONIA

OBJECTIVES

- To define cerebral palsy.
- To define dystonia.
- To discuss the treatment of dystonia.

VIGNETTE

A 19-year-old man with cerebral palsy developed tremulousness and abnormal posture of the head over the last year and a half.

CASE SUMMARY

This 19-year-old man has a history of microcephaly, developmental delay, static encephalopathy, spastic quadriparesis, and complex partial seizures with secondary generalization. Head imaging showed left hemispheric atrophy and diffuse ventricular enlargement and cerebellar atrophy. He has periods of head turning to the right likely representing a focal/cervical dystonia. He also shows a head tremor. He was treated with botulinum toxin injections into both sternocleidomastoid muscles, right and left splenius capitis muscles, left levator scapula, and right cervical trapezius.

Cerebral palsy is a static encephalopathy of prenatal or perinatal origin that affects motor tone and function, resulting in spasticity, hypotonia, ataxia, and dyskinesias. The diagnosis is made on a history of delayed motor milestones and on clinical examination. Intellectual impairment and seizures are fairly common. Dystonia is a disorder consisting of intermittent or sustained, often painful, twisting repetitive muscle spasms that may occur in one part of the body or throughout the entire body.

Cervical dystonia is often referred to as torticollis or spasmodic torticollis. It consists of intermittent uncontrollable spasms of neck muscles that is often associated with pain. It is the most common focal dystonia. It is often unilateral, ceases during sleep, and increases with stress or anxiety. Several abnormal head postures may occur (often in combination): rotation (torticollis), lateral tilt (laterocollis), hyperextension of the head (retrocollis), and forward flexion of the head (antecollis). Torticollis and laterocollis are the two most common head positions. By convention, spasmodic torticollis is named by the sternocleidomastoid that contracts.

Several medications can be used to treat dystonia such as anticholinergic medications, dopaminergic and antidopaminergic medications, benzodiazepines, some antidepressants, and some anticonvulsants. Perhaps one of the most effective and nontoxic treatments for focal dystonia is injection of botulinum toxin into the affected muscles. Side effects of botulinum toxin injections include excessive transient weakness of the injected muscle, dry mouth, and a local hematoma.

■ SELECTED REFERENCES

Biller J, ed. *Practical neurology,* 2nd ed. Philadelphia: Lippincott Williams & Wilkins, 2002.
Brashear A. The botulinum toxins and the treatment of cervical dystonia. *Semin Neurol* 2001;21:85–90.
Nass R. Developmental disabilities. In: Bradley WG, Daroff RB, Fenichel GM, et al., eds. *Neurology in clinical practice.* Philadelphia: Butterworth-Heineman, 2000:1585–1594.

■ SEE QUESTIONS: 189, 204

CASE 51

SPINAL MYOCLONUS/CARCINOMA OF THE OVARY

OBJECTIVES

- To present an example of segmental myoclonus of spinal cord origin.
- To discuss the differential diagnosis of spinal myoclonus.
- To summarize current management strategies for spinal myoclonus.

VIGNETTE

This 87-year-old woman was found to have a carcinoma of the ovary in 1997. She was treated surgically, and subsequently received chemotherapy with taxol and cis-platinum. After chemotherapy, she experienced numbness and tingling of her hands and feet as well as a loss of balance. She is consulting us now because of involuntary muscular spasms of her abdomen and involuntary contractions of her throat coming up from her diaphragm. These movements have affected her speech. The movements continue during the day but they seem to subside when sleeping. In June 2001 she fractured a rib and this has further aggravated her speech difficulty.

CASE SUMMARY

Our patient had painless, rhythmic, involuntary lower abdominal wall movements. The movements interfered with her voice and were not stimulus sensitive. The movements lessened during sleep. She had not received recent administration of epidural anesthesia or any diagnostic study involving the administration of intravenous contrast material. She did not have a history of recent dermatomal skin lesions or spine trauma. On examination, she had brief, rhythmic, and stereotyped involuntary contractions of both sides of her lower abdomen.

The jerks were spontaneous and not induced by tapping, flash, or sound. She did not have axial flexion or extension jerks, palatal myoclonus, contractions of the lower extremities, or pyramidal signs. Laboratory investigations (including paraneoplastic serology) and MRI of the spinal cord were unremarkable. Treatment with levetiracetam greatly diminished the frequency and amplitude of the myoclonic jerks with minimal side effects.

Our patient had hyperkinetic involuntary movements with the characteristics of spinal myoclonus. Spinal myoclonus is a rare movement disorder characterized by myoclonic involvement of a group of muscles supplied by a few contiguous segments of the spinal cord. Protracted myoclonic activity may rarely be the cause of rhabdomyolysis and myoglobinuria. The focal involuntary muscular contractions of spinal myoclonus have been associated with traumatic, infectious, inflammatory, ischemic, neoplastic, and degenerative lesions of the spinal cord.

Spinal myoclonus has been reported in association with spinal cord irradiation, spinal cord vascular malformations, Devic's disease, HTLV-1–associated myelopathy, paraneoplastic syndromes (paraneoplastic subacute motor neuronopathy), placement of epidural catheters, administration of interferon alpha treatment for hepatitis C, intravenous administration of iodine contrast media, chronic toluene intoxication, and in association with antibodies against glutamic acid decarboxylase. Spinal myoclonus has also been reported in association with brain death. Paraspinal myoclonus has been rarely found in association with root lesions.

Levetiracetam, clonazepam, or valproic acid alone or in combination with L-5 hydroxytryptophan have been used with varying success.

■ SELECTED REFERENCES

Brazis PW, Masdeu JC, Biller J. *Localization in clinical neurology,* 4th ed. Philadelphia: Lippincott Williams & Wilkins, 2001.
Fujimoto K, Yamauchi Y, Yoshida M. Spinal myoclonus in association with brain death. *Rinsho Shinkeigaku.* 1989;29:1417–1419.
Hoehn MM, Cherrington M. Spinal myoclonus. *Neurology* 1977;27:942–946.
Roobol TH, Kazzaz BA, Vecht CJ. Segmental rigidity and spinal myoclonus as a paraneoplastic syndrome. *J Neurol Neurosurg Psychiatry* 1987;50:628–631.

■ SEE QUESTIONS: 189, 228

CASE 52

PALATAL MYOCLONUS DUE TO MEDULLARY INFARCTION

OBJECTIVES

- To discuss the risk of recurrent strokes.
- To discuss palatal myoclonus (palatal tremor).
- To briefly review the main features of the medial medullary syndrome.

VIGNETTE

This 59-year-old man with a history of diabetes mellitus, hypertension, and prior CABG has had multiple strokes.

CASE SUMMARY

Our patient had multiple supratentorial and infratentorial ischemic strokes and was finally confined to a wheelchair due to his marked gait unsteadiness. Examination showed mild head titubation, dysarthria, asymmetric horizontal-torsional jerk nystagmus, and continuous rhythmic contractions affecting the palatal structures. He had no complaints of objective tinnitus or an ear click. MRI showed multiple supratentorial and infratentorial infarcts including a right medial medullary infarction. There was no appreciable hypertrophy of the inferior olivary nucleus. MRA did not show an ectatic vertebrobasilar system.

Every year, at least 750,000 Americans experience a new or recurrent stroke. Stroke remains the third leading cause of death, with approximately 165,000 stroke-related fatalities in the United States. Individuals with a history of cerebrovascular disease have increased risks of recurrent stroke, other cardiovascular events, and cognitive decline. Even silent brain infarcts increase the risk of developing dementia. It has been estimated that among stroke survivors, more than one-third have some form of long-term disability and one in six are likely to suffer a further stroke within 5 years.

Patients with a first stroke are at greater risk of recurrent stroke, especially, but not exclusively, early after the first stroke. Those who suffer a recurrent stroke have a higher mortality than patients with first stroke. If the recurrence is contralateral to the first stroke, prognosis for functional recovery is poor. The risk of stroke recurrence is increased also by the presence of underlying dementia.

Our patient had a constellation of clinical features including an asymmetric horizontal-torsional jerk nystagmus indicative of an abnormality of the vestibulocerebellar pathways. The continuous rhythmic contractions of his soft palate suggested the presence of palatal tremor formerly known as palatal myoclonus. Palatal myoclonus (palatal tremor) is a rare neurological condition characterized by continuous and synchronous contractions of the soft palate and other oropharyngeal muscles that occur at frequencies of 100 to 150 per minute (20 to 600). Concomitant contractions of other muscles including the larynx, extraocular muscles, neck, diaphragm, tongue and face may be observed.

Rarely, patients may complain of objective (audible both to the patient and to an observer) tinnitus or even dysphagia and respiratory difficulties. The condition is most often observed in adults and rarely in children. Palatal myoclonus comprises two separate disorders: essential palatal tremor, where ear clicking sounds are a prominent feature; and symptomatic palatal myoclonus, which is associated with cerebellar/brainstem disturbances. Palatal myoclonus is observed with lesions disrupting the pathway between the red nucleus, the inferior olivary nucleus, and the dentate nucleus (dentatorubroolivary pathway or Guillain-Mollaret triangle). The resulting denervation of the contralateral inferior olive leads to its hypertrophy.

Palatal myoclonus may result from cerebrovascular, demyelinating, neoplastic, encephalitic, postinfectious, neurodegenerative, or traumatic etiologies. Palatal myoclonus has also been associated to extrinsic compression of the inferior olive by an ectatic vertebral artery. An autosomal dominant form of palatal myoclonus with histopathologic features resembling Alexander's disease has been described. Palatal myoclonus is usually resistant to pharmacologic interventions. Baclofen, sodium valproate, clonazepam, benzodiazepines, lamotrigine, phenytoin, and piracetam have been attempted with variable results. Botulinum toxin injections have been used in an attempt to treat the objective tinnitus.

Our patient had multiple supratentorial and infratentorial ischemic infarcts. MRI shown on this video demonstrated a right medial medullary infarction. The medial medullary syndrome is less common than the lateral medullary syndrome, and it may be due to an occlusion of the vertebral artery, a branch of the vertebral artery, or the lower basilar artery. The findings with this syndrome include an ipsilateral lower motor neuron paralysis of the tongue (present in less than 30% to 50% of cases) and a contralateral paralysis of the arm and leg. In addition, there is contralateral hemibody loss of tactile, vibratory, and position sense.

■ **SELECTED REFERENCES**

Deuschl G, Mischke G, Schenck E, et al. Symptomatic and essential rhythmic palatal myoclonus. *Brain* 1990;113:1645–1672.
Meyer MA, David CE, Chahin NS. Palatal myoclonus secondary to vertebral artery compression of the inferior olive. *J Neuroimaging* 2000;10(Oct):221–223.
Okamoto Y, Mitsuyama H, Jonosono M, et al. Autosomal dominant palatal myoclonus and spinal cord atrophy. *J Neurol Sci* 2002;195(Mar 15):71–76.
Wolfe C. The impact of stroke. *Br Med Bull* 2000;56:275–286.

■ **SEE QUESTIONS: 47, 50, 88**

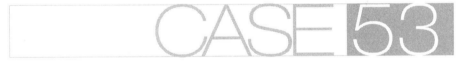

LACUNAR HEMICHOREOATHETOSIS

OBJECTIVE

▓ To demonstrate a hyperkinetic presentation of a lacunar stroke.

VIGNETTE

This 56-year-old woman with a history of hypertension had the sudden onset of paresthesias on her whole left side including face, trunk, and both extremities. In the following minutes to hours, she developed weakness of her left upper extremity. She also developed some weakness of the left lower extremity. Since then, she has been left with some weakness mostly of the distal left upper extremity as well as a mild gait difficulty. She has also developed adventitious movements on her left upper extremity.

CASE SUMMARY

Our patient had a history of uncontrolled arterial hypertension. She abruptly developed left hemibody numbness and mild weakness. This was followed by random jerking, involuntary movements of her left hand and arm. Some degree of a persistent posture in overflexion and overextension was also observed. The movements disappeared during sleep. She did not have any facial grimacing or tongue protrusion. MRI showed a lacunar infarction of the contralateral putamen and caudate nuclei with sparing of the anterior limb of the internal capsule. Random blood sugar and thyroid function tests were normal. Additional ancillary investigations for the presence of antiphospholipid antibodies or polycythemia were unremarkable.

Ischemic strokes may result from (i) large artery atherosclerotic disease, (ii) small vessel or penetrating artery disease (lacunes), (iii) cardiogenic embolism, (iv) nonatherosclerotic vasculopathies, (v) hypercoagulable disorders, and (vi) infarcts of undetermined cause. Lacunar infarcts involve deep regions of the brain or brainstem. The most frequent sites of involvement are the putamen, basis pontis, thalamus, posterior limb of the internal capsule, and caudate nucleus. Multiple lacuna are associated strongly with arterial hypertension and diabetes mellitus. Lacunar infarcts are often associated with *in situ* occlusion of a single perforating vessel or thickening of the arteriolar wall.

Lacunar infarcts have a relatively favorable prognosis as they are usually associated with a good functional recovery, a lower recurrence rate, and a higher survival rate than other types of ischemic strokes. Although there are over twenty described lacunar syndromes, those that have been best described are pure motor hemiparesis (PMH), pure sensory stroke (PSS), sensorimotor stroke (SMS), ataxic hemiparesis (AH), and dysarthria clumsy hand syndrome (DCHS). Hemichorea/hemiballismus (HH), the most frequently reported movement disorder associated with acute stroke, is an uncommon presentation of a lacunar infarction. Some degree of dystonia and athetosis may be present as well.

Discrete ischemic or hemorrhagic lesions of the basal ganglia may be associated with contralateral hyperkinetic motor activity confined to one side of the body (hemichorea or hemiballismus). Lesions in or near the subthalamic nucleus produce contralateral hemiballismus. Hemiballismus may also result from lesions in the caudate, putamen, globus pallidus, precentral gyrus, or thalamic nuclei. Destruction of the pyramidal tract ipsilateral to the subthalamic nucleus prevents the development of hemiballismus. Small unilateral lesions of the anteroventral portion of the caudate cause contralateral choreoathetosis. Unilateral lesions of the globus pallidus may cause contralateral hemidystonia. Unilateral pallidal-putaminal lesions may present with sudden falling to the contralateral side while sitting, standing, or walking.

Repetitive involuntary movements (hemichorea and hemiballismus) have been reported with lacunar infarction of the basal ganglia and with carotid artery occlusive disease. Hemichorea and hemiballismus have also been reported in older women in association with nonketotic hyperglycemia. Uncommonly, involuntary tonic spasms of a limb may occur with brainstem lacunar infarctions. Focal hand dystonia has been observed in patients with lacunar infarctions of the lenticular or caudate nucleus, whereas posthemiplegic athetosis may develop after ischemic or hemorrhagic lesions of the contralateral putamen and to a variable extent the globus pallidus.

■ SELECTED REFERENCES

Ghika J, Bogousslavsky J. Abnormal movements. In: Bogousslavsky J, Caplan L, eds. *Stroke syndromes.* Cambridge, UK: Cambridge University Press, 1995:91–101.

Kase CS, Maulsby GO, de Juan E, et al. Hemichorea-hemiballism and lacunar infarction in the basal ganglia. *Neurology* 1981;31:452–455.

Kaufman DK, Brown RD, Karnes WE. Involuntary tonic spasms of a limb due to a brainstem lacunar infarction. *Stroke* 1994;25:217–219.

Lee B-C, Hwang S-H, Chang GY. Hemiballismus-hemichorea in older diabetic women: a clinical syndrome with MRI correlation. *Neurology* 1999;52:646–648.

■ SEE QUESTIONS: 189, 200

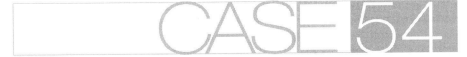

PARANEOPLASTIC CHOREA/SENSORY NEURONOPATHY

OBJECTIVE

▓ To review the causes of sensory neuronopathy and outline an appropriate diagnostic evaluation.

VIGNETTE

A 63-year-old retired coal miner initially had pain in the left upper extremity and then began to develop burning and numbness as well as weakness in both upper extremities. The left upper extremity has remained worse than the right. The patient has not noticed problems in his legs. Currently the patient has trouble eating, he cannot hold onto a fork, he cannot tie his shoes, and he cannot clean his dentures because of difficulty manipulating objects with his hands. He cannot drive adequately because he does not feel that he has good control of the steering wheel. He cannot write secondary to trouble holding a pen.

CASE SUMMARY

The patient presents with a striking combination of sensory disturbance in the limbs that has progressed slowly over time, involving primarily large fiber sensory dysfunction. In addition, the patient has involuntary movements of the hands and face that resemble chorea.

Regarding localization of the sensory neuropathy and neuronopathy, most distal sensory peripheral neuropathies have symptoms beginning in the feet initially, then eventually spreading to the hands. Most symptoms involve small sensory fibers dealing with pain and temperature initially or predominantly. There are a few sensory peripheral neuropathies that tend to begin with symmetric symptoms in the upper extremities, then secondarily spread to the lower extremities; these tend to be conditions that affect the dorsal root ganglia or nerve roots as opposed to more distal aspects of the nerve.

A list of such sensory neuropathies or neuronopathies that affect the dorsal root ganglia and that may affect the arms early would include the following: toxic neuropathies that affect the dorsal root ganglia such as vincristine or cisplatin neuropathy, vitamin B_6 or pyridoxine toxicity, the sensory findings and symptoms of subacute combined system degeneration from vitamin B_{12} deficiency, Sjögren's sensory neuronopathy, autoimmune or postinfectious polyradiculopathy or sensory ganglionopathy (in other words, a sensory form of Guillain-Barré syndrome), and a paraneoplastic sensory neuronopathy associated with anti-Hu antibody as a remote effect of malignancy.

The second localization issue is whether or not the patient actually has the problem in the peripheral nerve at all or whether it is more likely a spinal cord lesion involving the dorsal columns. A compressive myelopathy, syringomyelia, cord tumor, myelitis or sarcoid affecting the cord, as well as multiple sclerosis are all worth considering as possible causes of a myelopathy in such patients.

The management of sensory neuronopathy in a patient with paraneoplastic syndrome can be difficult. As with most of the paraneoplastic syndromes, the primary goal is the successful treatment of the underlying malignancy. Therefore, if the primary tumor can be detected, then that should be the first strategy for management. A number of paraneoplastic syndromes are successfully treated when the malignancy is resolved, such as Lambert-Eaton syndrome. The second strategy for treatment would be immunotherapy in the view that if the disorder is antibody mediated, control of antibody production may help the patient's symptomatology.

This approach applies to the broad spectrum of paraneoplastic syndromes, and there is a variable degree of improvement with this form of therapy depending on the syndrome. In this particular patient, we would favor using plasmapheresis, although i.v. Ig would be another alternative.

With regard to the patient's movement disorder, it is rare to have chorea as a remote affect of malignancy, and a search for an underlying occult cancer is not usually central to the workup of a new patient with isolated chorea. However, chorea as part of a paraneoplastic syndrome has been reported, including those with anti-CRMP-5 antibodies (IgG), which may be detected in serum and in spinal fluid in association with chest malignancy (small cell lung cancer 80% and occasionally thymoma).

■ **SELECTED REFERENCE**

Biller J, ed. *Practical neurology,* 2nd ed. Philadelphia: Lippincott Williams & Wilkins, 2002.

■ **SEE QUESTIONS: 186, 189, 200, 228, 230, 241**

CASE 55

HEMIFACIAL SPASM

OBJECTIVES

- To present an example of sporadic idiopathic hemifacial spasm.
- To discuss the differential diagnosis of unilateral involuntary facial movements.
- To summarize current management strategies for hemifacial spasm.

VIGNETTE

A 69-year-old man has had brief painless twitches around the right eye and also around the right corner of his mouth for the last year. Sometimes the twitches are so intense that they narrow his right palpebral fissure. He has had no previous facial palsy or facial trauma. He has no tinnitus, vertigo, or disequilibrium.

CASE SUMMARY

This tape was obtained after treatment was initiated. Our patient had an insidious onset of brief, painless, unilateral clonic contractions of the facial musculature beginning in the orbicularis oculi that gradually progressed downward to involve other facial muscles. The facial contractions were exacerbated by anxiety and fatigue. His wife had noted that the movements persisted during sleep. He had no history of Bell's palsy or traumatic facial injury. MRI and MRA were unremarkable. A diagnosis of sporadic idiopathic hemifacial spasm was made. The patient received botulinum toxin injections to the involved muscles.

Hemifacial spasm has been classically ascribed to vascular loop compression of the facial nerve at the root exit zone from the pons. Causes other than vascular loops include tortuous basilar artery, vertebral artery dolichoectasia, vertebrobasilar junction dissecting aneurysms, cerebellopontine angle mass lesions, Paget's disease of the bone, idiopathic intracranial hypertension, and parotid gland tumors. Hemifacial spasm may also follow Bell's palsy or traumatic facial nerve injuries (postparalytic hemifacial spasm).

Bilateral hemifacial spasm is unusual; the contractions are usually asymmetric and asynchronus. Hemifacial spasm is seldom found in children or adolescents. Pediatric hemifacial spasm may be due to an underlying intracranial tumor. Rare cases of familial hemifacial spasm have been reported, but most cases are sporadic. Hemifacial spasm should be differentiated from other conditions including facial dystonia, blepharospasm, facial myokymia, facial tics, hemimasticastory spasm, paretic facial contracture, tardive dyskinesia, and psychogenic facial spasm.

Relief of hemifacial spasm may occur with botulinum toxin injection or with microvascular decompression. 3D-TOF MRA can identify the vascular compression of the exit zone of the facial nerve and assist in preoperative planning. MR cisternography is valuable in identifying the blood vessels and nerve bundles in the cerebellopontine cistern. Gabapentin, carbamazepine, clonazepam, phenytoin, and levodopa/carbidopa may be useful in some patients with hemifacial spasm.

■ SELECTED REFERENCES

Brazis PW, Masdeu JC, Biller J. *Localization in clinical neurology,* 4th ed. Philadelphia: Lippincott Williams & Wilkins, 2001.

Samii M, Gunther T, Iaconetta G, et al. Microvascular decompression to treat hemifacial spasm: long-term results for a consecutive series of 143 patients. *Neurosurgery* 2002;50:712–718.

Wang A, Jankovic J. Hemifacial spasm: clinical correlates and treatments. *Muscle Nerve* 1998;21:1740–1747.

■ SEE QUESTION: 152

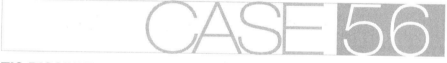

TIC DISORDER

OBJECTIVES

■ To discuss the clinical classification of tics.
■ To review the spectrum of clinical disorders associated with tics.
■ To briefly review the clinical characteristics and management of Tourette syndrome (TS).

VIGNETTE

A 38-year-old man was referred for evaluation of head shaking and shoulder twitches. He had head shaking and shoulder twitches early on in childhood but did not seek medical attention until about 10 years ago. He states that being home alone decreases his abnormal head and shoulder twitches. He has no head or shoulder twitches during sleep. Taking hot baths also makes his twitches better.

CASE SUMMARY

Our patient presented with a long history of brief intermittent stereotyped, purposeless, and irregularly repetitive clonic hyperkinesias consistent with a motor tic disorder. He also had a history of a generalized anxiety disorder. The motor tics initially became noticeable in grade school with persistent throat clearing and blinking. In middle and high school, these symptoms worsened. They now also included simple motor movements like head shaking and shoulder shrugging. The throat clearing has since dissipated. He had no grunting or barking. He described the period before the tics as consisting of an initial buildup of tension, which the tic then relieved. The symptoms have worsened within the previous year. They occur with greater intensity, but not significantly reduced frequency, when he is at home and relaxed.

He works the night shift at his job, but he prefers to work at home as he feels less anxious there. Although the absence of other workers during the night shift helps anxiety, the thought of pending incomplete work makes him nervous. He also sits in the back of movies and at church as he is embarrassed about his symptoms. He had no ritualistic thoughts surrounding the tics nor intrusive, uncontrollable, or recurrent thoughts. He did not describe any compulsive behaviors, such as hand washing or need for organization. Other than throat clearing, there have never been phonic tics.

His symptoms of anxiety include worrying all the time, having different thoughts about different daily issues, shakiness, some problems with concentration, and feeling panicky and overwhelmed at times. The patient also thought that the motor tic disorder contributed toward some of the anxiety.

He had been placed on haloperidol, but this caused severe incoordination and was discontinued. He also tried carbamazepine, baclofen, and depakote, which had no effect. Cranial computed tomography (CT) and EEG were normal. Our patient had some modest control of the tics with clonazepam.

Examination showed an awake, alert, and well-oriented man who provided his own history in good detail. He was neatly dressed. He was cheery and his affect reactive. He had good insight into his illness including the tic disorder and anxiety. No hallucinations or delusions were present. There was no psychomotor agitation or retardation. Thoughts were well organized, logical, and goal oriented. The patient had simple motor tics, about three to four tics every minute. The tics were mostly in the region of the shoulders and head. Obvious motor disturbances included frequent head twisting and jerking and shoulder shrugging, left greater than right. There were no coprolalia, echolalia, hiccoughs, or other associated vocal disturbances.

His fund of general knowledge was average for his age and reading was low average. Speech was fluent without dysarthria or aphasia. Digit span was normal. Visual motor scanning speed was intact. Novel problem solving was largely normal. Immediate recall was average. Learning with rehearsal was low normal. Long-term recall was average. Visual confrontation naming was normal. Constructional praxis was intact.

The Personality Assessment Inventory was primarily remarkable for mild symptoms of anxiety. The remainder of his neurological examination was unremarkable.

Our clinical diagnosis was motor tic disorder and generalized anxiety disorder. Tics may present suddenly or gradually and may have spontaneous remissions. Tics are characterized by brief, rapid, usually stereotyped, purposeless, irregularly repetitive, and predominantly clonic hyperkinesias involving one or more muscular groups. Tics may consist of simple motor movements (e.g., eye blinking, nose twitch, shoulder shrug, head jerking), complex motor movements (e.g., head shaking, skipping), simple phonic sounds (e.g., throat clearing, grunting, barking), or complex vocalizations (e.g., coprolalia, echolalia, palilalia, hiccoughs).

Besides temporary suppressibility, premonitory urge, and stereotypic appearance, tics may be exacerbated with stress, excitement, boredom, and fatigue. Tics have been clinically classified into the following: (i) simple motor tics (clonic, dystonic, or tonic), (ii) complex motor tics (seemingly purposeful or seemingly nonpurposeful), (iii) simple phonic tics, (iv) complex phonic tics, and (v) compulsive tics. There is also a transient tic syndrome of childhood, where the tics may occur for no longer than 12 consecutive months.

Tics may occur secondary to drugs (L-dopa, neuroleptics, methylphenidate, carbamazepine, phenytoin, phenobarbital, lamotrigine) or striatal disorders (e.g., neuroacanthocytosis; Huntington disease; Sydenham chorea; Wilson's disease; primary dystonia; encephalitis lethargica; posttraumatic, poststroke, after carbon monoxide poisoning), frontal lobe degenerations, Creutzfeldt-Jakob disease, and may also occur in Tourette syndrome (TS). TS is a sporadic or inherited complex neuropsychiatric syndrome with onset in childhood (before age 18) and thought to be related to hyperactive basal ganglia thalamocortical pathways. Inheritance of TS may involve autosomal dominant, bilinear, or polygenic mechanisms.

TS is characterized by multiple or single motor tics (e.g., nose twitching, blinking, neck or shoulder movements), often associated with vocalization (grunting, sniffling, snorting, barking, throat clearing, spitting, coughing) or occasionally with more complicated motor activity, such as copropraxia (obscene gesturing), echopraxia (imitations of acts), jumping, or kicking. Coprolalia (obscene language), copropraxia (obscene gesturing), and echolalia (tendency to repeat words or sentences recently spoken to the patient) occur in less than one-third or one-half of affected individuals. Some patients may experience intrusive coprolalic thoughts (i.e., mental coprolalia) or exhibit coprographia.

The tics of Tourette syndrome may have a waxing and waning course and are often accompanied by behavioral problems, such as obsessive-compulsive disorder (OCD), attention deficit hyperactivity disorder (ADHD), other anxiety disorders, disruptive behavior disorders, learning disabilities, and school problems. Coprolalia may also occur with Lesch-Nyhan syndrome, postencephalitic parkinsonism, choreoacanthocytosis, and other basal ganglia disorders. Adult-onset tic disorders may be caused by infection, trauma, cocaine use, or neuroleptic exposure, or may be idiopathic. Childhood tic disorders have been associated with group A β-hemolytic streptococcal infections and termed PANDAS (pediatric autoimmune neuropsychiatric disorders associated with streptococcus).

Treatment may be difficult. Given the high frequency of psychiatric comorbidity, complete elimination of the tics is no longer the primary goal of therapy. Timely and accurate diagnosis and education of the patient and family are essential elements of effective management. A large variety of pharmacologic agents are now available to treat patients with tics, including neuroleptics, dopamine anatagonists, clonidine, reserpine, tetrabenazine, guanfacine, clonazepam, trazodone, verapamil, deprenyl, pergolide, nicotine, and botulinum toxin injections (for dystonic tics). Plasma exchange and intravenous immunoglobulin (i.v. IG) has been used in children with infection-triggered tic disorder and obsessive compulsive disorder.

■ SELECTED REFERENCES

Biller J, ed. *Practical neurology,* 2nd ed. Philadelphia: Lippincott Williams & Wilkins, 2002.

Brazis PW, Masdeu JC, Biller J. *Localization in clinical neurology,* 4th ed. Philadelphia: Lippincott Williams & Wilkins, 2001.

Perlmutter SJ, Leitman SF, Garvey MA, et al. Therapeutic plasma exchange and intravenous immunoglobulin for obsessive-compulsive disorder and tic disorders in childhood. *Lancet* 1999;354:1137–1138.

Shapiro AK, Shapiro ES, Young JG, et al., eds. Gilles de la Tourette syndrome, 2nd ed. New York: Raven Press, 1988.

■ SEE QUESTIONS: 44, 189

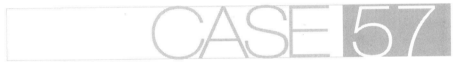

HEMIDYSTONIA (SARCOIDOSIS)

OBJECTIVES

■ To emphasize the rarity of sarcoidosis exclusively manifested by hemidystonia.
■ To discuss lesion localization in cases of hemidystonia.
■ To briefly review the major neurological manifestations of sarcoidosis.

VIGNETTE

This 34-year-old man was diagnosed with sarcoidosis by biopsy of a lymph node in the inguinal area around 1 year prior to presentation. He presented to the neurology clinic after rapid onset of involuntary movements of the left arm that were mainly proximal and present with action. Over time, his involuntary movements have extended to affect the left side of his neck, left side of his face, and to a lesser extent his trunk and left leg.

CASE SUMMARY

Our patient had biopsy-proven sarcoidosis and presented with a hyperkinetic movement disorder suggestive of hemidystonia. Most patients with hemidystonia have neuroimaging evidence of contralateral basal ganglia lesions. Hemidystonia may follow lesions in the contralateral caudate, lentiform nucleus (especially the putamen), or thalamus, or a combination of these structures. Hemidystonia may be caused by abnormal input from the thalamus to the premotor cortex due to lesions either of the thalamus itself or of the striatum projecting by way of the globus pallidus to the thalamus. Lesions associated with dystonic spasms or myoclonic dystonia tend to be located in the striatopallidal complex or thalamus contralateral to the dystonia. Paroxysmal hemidystonia may occur with contralateral midbrain lesions. Besides stroke and head trauma, other causes of hemidystonia include encephalitis, vascular malformations, porencephalic cysts, thalamotomy, and a variety of neurodegenerative disorders.

Sarcoidosis is a chronic multisystem granulomatous disease characterized by noncaseating granulomatous reaction of unknown origin. It most frequently involves the lymph nodes and lungs, but any organ can be involved. Sarcoidosis occurs most commonly in adults 20 to 40 years old. It is more common in women than in men, and in the United States, African-Americans are more commonly affected than whites. Involvement of the nervous system represents 5% to 15% of cases.

Major neurological manifestations of sarcoidosis include cranial neuropathies (most commonly the facial nerve), encephalopathy, aseptic chronic or recurrent basilar meningitis (sometimes associated with borderline low CSF glucose levels), diabetes insipidus, brain mass, seizures, angiopathy (vasculitis/vasculopathy), hydrocephalus, basal ganglia dysfunction, myelopathy, polyneuropathy, mononeuritis multiplex, and acute and chronic myopathy. The triad of parotitis, uveitis, and facial nerve palsy is known as Heerfordt's syndrome. Hemidystonia as a manifestation of CNS sarcoidosis is extraordinarily uncommon.

The clinical course of sarcoidosis is highly variable including exacerbations and spontaneous remissions. The mainstay of treatment is corticosteroids. Cyclosporine may be useful in cases of refractory neurosarcoidosis.

■ SELECTED REFERENCES

Brazis PW, Masdeu JC, Biller J. *Localization in clinical neurology,* 4th ed. Philadelphia: Lippincott Williams & Wilkins, 2001.

Delaney P. Neurologic manifestations of sarcoidosis. Review of the literature with a report of 23 cases. *Ann Intern Med* 1977;87:336–346.

Fahn S, Bressman S, Marsden CD. Classification of dystonia. *Adv Neurol* 1998;78:1–10.

Stern BJ, Krumholz A, Johns C, et al. Sarcoidosis and its neurological manifestations. *Arch Neurol* 1985;42:909–917.

■ SEE QUESTIONS: 190, 204, 234, 240

CASE 58

ACUTE DYSTONIC REACTION

OBJECTIVES

- To illustrate a neurologic complication of a dopamine receptor blocking agent.
- To review management guidelines of neuroleptic-induced acute dystonic reactions.

VIGNETTE

This 41-year-old woman with systemic lupus erythematous, IgM anticardiolipin antibody, and branch retinal vein occlusion of the right eye had a history of what she labeled as "an allergic reaction" to Compazine following abdominal surgery.

CASE SUMMARY

Our patient suffered an acute dystonic reaction induced by prochlorperazine (Compazine). Neurologic complications of dopamine receptor blocking agents include acute dystonic reactions, acute akathisia, neuroleptic malignant syndrome, neuroleptic-induced parkinsonism including the "rabbit syndrome," and tardive dyskinesia. Acute dystonic reactions are motor side effects that occur within the first few days after the initiation of neuroleptic treatment. Most frequently, acute neuroleptic-induced acute dystonia involves the muscles of the face, tongue, jaw, neck, or throat. The most typical signs involve oculogyric crisis, trismus, and opisthotonic posturing. A rarely reported extrapyramidal reaction is acute laryngeal dystonia (laryngospasm).

Risk factors for acute dystonic reactions include young age, male gender (particularly African-American and Asian-American men), and use of high potency neuroleptics (e.g., haloperidol, fluphenazine). Parenteral administration of 2 mg benztropine (Cogentin) or 50 mg diphenhydramine (Benadryl) are the most effective medications in the majority of cases, but prophylactic use of oral anticholinergics should be continued as outpatient therapy for 48 to 72 hours. Intravenous administration of anticholinergics usually relieves symptoms within 2 to 3 minutes, whereas intramuscular administration requires approximately 15 to 30 minutes for symptom relief. Geriatric patients generally require lower doses of anticholinergic drugs. Phencyclidine (PCP) exposure should be suspected in cases of acute dystonic reactions failing to respond to diphenhydramine.

■ SELECTED REFERENCES

Brazis PW, Masdeu JC, Biller J. *Localization in clinical neurology*, 4th ed. Philadelphia: Lippincott Williams & Wilkins, 2001.

Fahn S, Bressman S, Marsden CD. Classification of dystonia. *Adv Neurol* 1998;78:1–10.

Koek RJ, Pi EH. Acute laryngeal dystonic reactions to neuroleptics. *Psychosomatics* 1990;31:236–237.

Piecuch S, Thomas U, Shah BR. Acute dystonic reactions that fail to respond to diphenhydramine: think of PCP. *J Emerg Med* 2000;18:379–381.

■ **SEE QUESTIONS: 108, 204**

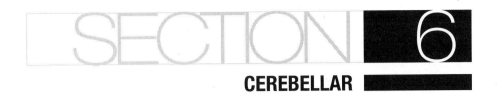

SECTION 6

CEREBELLAR

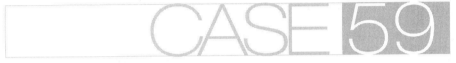

CASE 59

ATAXIA DUE TO BILATERAL PICA INFARCTIONS

OBJECTIVES

- To highlight the cardinal features of cerebellar dysfunction.
- To review the arterial supply of the cerebellum.
- To discuss the clinical presentation and management of large cerebellar infarcts.

VIGNETTE

This 47-year-old man had a right cerebellar hemispherectomy secondary to a large cerebellar stroke (bilateral PICA infarcts, right greater than left).

CASE SUMMARY

Our patient was a previously healthy 47-year-old man who had sudden onset of shortness of breath, nausea, diaphoresis, disequilibrium, and dysarthria. He was admitted to another hospital and was diagnosed to have a myocardial infarction and a stroke. A 2D echocardiogram showed an ejection fraction of 55% and no intracavitary thrombi. MRI of the brain showed bilateral posterior inferior cerebellar artery (PICA) territory infarctions. A cerebral angiogram showed an occluded right vertebral artery and near occlusion of the left vertebral artery. During the angiographic procedure, he had neurologic decline with disconjugate gaze and bradycardia.

The hospital course was complicated by obstructive hydrocephalus requiring drain and subsequent resection of cerebellar necrotic tissue. He also developed heparin-induced thrombocytopenia and was treated with plasmapheresis and

Refludan. Since hospital discharge, he has had no recurrent TIAs or strokes and was wheelchair bound and unable to walk due to marked ataxia. A follow-up MRA of the vertebrobasilar circulation showed complete recanalization of the vertebral arteries. He was diagnosed with polycythemia rubra vera.

Cardinal features of cerebellar dysfunction involve disturbances in motor control, muscle tone regulation, and coordination of skilled movements. As shown in the tape, the salient neurological findings in our patient were ataxia of the limbs and trunk, gait with dysmetria on finger-to-nose and heel-knee-shin testing, dysdiadochokinesia, and an impaired checking response. Speech was scanning and slurred, typical of cerebellar dysarthria. He also had a wide-based stance and gait and initially could not ambulate as he was falling in any direction.

The arterial supply of the cerebellum is provided by the posterior inferior cerebellar artery (PICA), the anterior inferior cerebellar artery (AICA), and the superior cerebellar artery (SCA). The PICA branches from the vertebral artery, whereas AICA and SCA branch from the basilar artery. The PICA encircles the medulla to supply the lateral medulla. The distal portions of PICA bifurcate into a medial trunk that supplies the vermis and the adjacent cerebellar hemisphere and a lateral trunk that supplies the cortical surface of the tonsil and cerebellar hemisphere. The AICA supplies the lateral tegmentum of the lower two-thirds of the pons and the ventrolateral cerebellum. The internal auditory artery arises from AICA to supply the facial and auditory nerves. The SCA supplies the superolateral cerebellar hemispheres, the superior cerebellar peduncle, the dentate nucleus, and part of the middle cerebellar peduncle.

Cerebellar infarctions usually result from thrombotic or embolic occlusion of a long circumferential cerebellar vessel and can be caused by a variety of disorders. Cerebellar arterial occlusions often result from cardioembolism, embolism from a vertebral artery plaque, or local arterial thrombosis. The infarctions may be limited to the cerebellum or may involve the brainstem or other structures. Four types of cerebellar infarction are recognized corresponding to the arterial territories of (i) PICA, (ii) AICA, (iii) SCA, and (iv) the cortical watershed and deep cerebellar white matter border-zone infarcts.

Cerebellar infarction typically presents with severe vertigo, nausea, vomiting, and ataxia. Loss of balance and difficulty maintaining posture, standing, and walking should suggest the presence of cerebellar disease. With large or bilateral cerebellar infarcts, the edematous cerebellum may compress the aqueduct of Sylvius or the fourth ventricle, causing acute obstructive hydrocephalus, or may compress the brainstem, resulting in a decreased level of alertness. With a cerebellar pressure cone, there is downward displacement of the cerebellar tonsils through the foramen magnum, resulting in neck stiffness, cardiac and respiratory rhythm disturbances, apnea, and death.

With upward transtentorial herniation, there is upward displacement of the superior aspect of the cerebellar hemisphere through the edge of the tentorial incisura, resulting in midbrain compression. Clinical manifestations of upward cerebellar herniation include lethargy, coma, paralysis of upward gaze, midposition and unreactive pupils, and abnormal extensor posturing.

Patients with cerebellar infarction should be admitted to an intensive care unit or a dedicated stroke unit. Large cerebellar infarcts tend to involve the territory of

PICA, SCA, or both. Emergency surgery (e.g., ventriculostomy or posterior fossa decompression or both) is often required.

■ SELECTED REFERENCES

Brazis PW, Masdeu JC, Biller J. *Localization in clinical neurology,* 4th ed. Philadelphia: Lippincott Williams & Wilkins, 2001.
Caplan LR. *Stroke: a clinical approach.* Boston: Butterworth-Heineman, 2000.
Heros RC. Cerebellar hemorrhage and infarction. *Stroke* 1982;13:106–109.
Love BB, Biller J. Neurovascular system. In: Goetz CG, ed. *Textbook of clinical neurology,* 2nd ed. WB Saunders, 2003.

■ SEE QUESTIONS: 19, 92, 143, 183

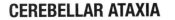

CASE 60

CEREBELLAR ATAXIA

OBJECTIVES

▨ To review the clinical presentation of midline cerebellar dysfunction.
▨ To outline the differential diagnosis of acquired progressive cerebellar degeneration and summarize the appropriate laboratory evaluation.

VIGNETTE

Seven years ago, this 75-year-old woman was just about to descend some concrete steps when she hesitated because she felt that her balance was off. Since then, she has noticed she felt a need to hold onto the rails or walls for support. Sometimes she made sure that both feet were on one step at the same time, but in doing so she still felt that she was rocking back and forth.

CASE SUMMARY

This 75-year-old woman has a 7-year history of slowly progressive ataxia with mild sensory loss and downbeat nystagmus. Finger-to-nose testing showed a very mild intention tremor, left greater than right, but no dysmetria. Heel-shin testing was mildly abnormal bilaterally. Rapid alternating movements were decreased bilaterally. Sensory examination showed decreased sensation to pinprick in the bilateral symmetric distal distribution in the hands and feet. When she attempted to stand, she had a very wide based stance and could not stand unassisted. She uses a walker to ambulate.

The differential diagnosis for progressive cerebellar ataxia can be grouped into hereditary causes and acquired causes. The hereditary causes include not only the spectrum of spinocerebellar ataxias (SCA) but also vitamin E deficiency, abetalipoproteinemia, ataxia telangiectasia, adrenoleukodystrophy, ataxia with Co-Q deficiency, late-onset G_{M2} gangliosidoses, mitochondrial diseases, sialidosis, maple syrup urine disease, organic acidurias, and cerebrotendinous xanthomatosis (CTX), Refsum's disease, Wilson's disease, and Niemann-Pick type C as examples. Although many of these disorders can be ruled out on clinical grounds, some of them require laboratory screening, especially those with therapeutic implications (CTX is treatable with chenodeoxycholic acid, vitamin E deficiency responds to high-dose vitamin E, etc.).

Acquired causes of progressive ataxia include paraneoplastic cerebellar degeneration. In women with subacute progressive ataxia, a thorough search for ovarian cancer is essential. Anti-Yo (anti-Purkinje cell) antibodies are typically present in the serum of such patients. Less commonly patients with malignancy will develop cerebellar ataxia and associate anti-Hu, anti-Ri, anti-Ta, or anti-Ma antibodies. Ethanol toxicity should be considered as should thiamine deficiency. Elderly patients are prone to a poor diet, especially those who live alone. Thiamine deficiency should be considered in any patient presenting with unexplained ataxia.

Multiple sclerosis, posterior fossa tumor, vascular disease, and craniovertebral junction lesions (such as Chiari malformation) are relatively easy to diagnose based on the combination of clinical presentation and MRI. Hypothyroidism is a rare cause of cerebellar ataxia, as is B_{12} deficiency. Toxins other than alcohol include phenytoin, chemotherapy, solvents such as toluene, and heavy metals (mercury). Infections such as CJD should be considered. Immune-mediated cerebellar degeneration (other than paraneoplastic) includes a form seen with anti-GAD antibodies and a gluten ataxia seen with antigliadin and antiendomysial antibodies.

This patient's MRI has shown atrophy of the anterosuperior vermis. She has had negative anti-Hu antibodies and negative anti-Purkinje cell antibodies. She has had normal immunoelectrophoresis, very long chain fatty acids and phytanic acid, and ammonia. She has had a negative porphyrin screen. She has had normal plasma cholestanol. Thyroid-stimulating hormone (TSH) and vitamin E are normal. She has had testing for SCA 1, 2, 3, 6, and 7 which were normal. She has also had normal testing for Friedreich's ataxia as well as DRPLA. Her B_{12} level has been below normal and she is therefore taking B_{12} injections. Patients with unexplained progressive cerebellar degeneration should be given an empirical trial of high-dose vitamin E.

■ **SELECTED REFERENCES**

Posner J, Dalmau JO. Paraneoplastic syndromes of the nervous system. *Clin Chem Lab Med* 2000;38:117–122.

Saiz A, Arpa J, Sagasta A, et al. Autoantibodies to glutamic acid decarboxylase in three patients with cerebellar ataxia, late-onset insulin-dependent diabetes mellitus, and polyendocrine autoimmunity. *Neurology* 1997;49:1026–1030.

Selim M, Drachman DA. Ataxia associated with Hashimoto's disease: progressive non-familial adult onset cerebellar degeneration with autoimmune thyroiditis. *J Neurol Neurosurg Psychiatry* 2001;71(Jul): 81–87.

Verino S, Lennon VA. New Purkinje cell antibody (PCA-2): marker of lung cancer-related neurological autoimmunity. *Ann Neurol* 2000;47:297–305.

■ SEE QUESTIONS: 42, 85, 143, 241

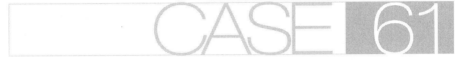

HEREDITARY ATAXIA

OBJECTIVES

▧ To review the clinical features of hereditary ataxia.
▧ To outline distinctive clinical features in the subtypes of spinocerebellar ataxia (SCA).

VIGNETTE

A 31-year-old woman had a progressive history of gait and limb incoordination and head tremors.

CASE SUMMARY

This woman presented with a 4-year history of progressive ataxia beginning in her early 20s. Her family history is positive, suggesting a dominant pattern of inheritance (with age of onset in the 20s). She has had diplopia, sensory loss, and tremor as prominent early features. Frequent headaches complicate her course.

Neurologic examination reveals severe dysarthria. Extraocular movements were abnormal, showing a left esotropia. She has marked head and hand tremor. Muscle stretch reflexes are hypoactive. The gait is severely wide based and ataxic. This patient appears to have a hereditary spinocerebellar ataxia (SCA) with a dominant pattern of inheritance.

SCA 1 begins with gait ataxia, and over time patients develop severe dysarthria and dysphagia. Ophthalmoparesis, spasticity, and choreoathetosis are common associated symptoms. Most patients become wheelchair bound within 15 years of the clinical onset of ataxia. These patients resemble those described in the past as having olivopontocerebellar atrophy. SCA 3 (Machado-Joseph disease) is the most common dominantly inherited ataxia in the world. The clinical picture varies but usually involves progressive ataxia along with abnormalities of eye movements, speech, and swallowing. Onset is typically in the 30s or 40s but occasionally patients present as late as age 60. Most patients develop some degree of supranuclear ophthalmoparesis. Facial myokymia (resembling fasciculations) is common.

Peripheral neuropathy, dystonia, parkinsonism, and motor neuron disease may occur. SCA 2, 3, and 6 are among the more common of the dominantly inherited ataxias. SCA 6 is typically milder in its clinical manifestations. Patients often have mild sensory loss. The clinical course is relatively slow. SCA 7 is associated with retinal degeneration. SCA 8 test results are more problematic as some individuals have a very large SCA 8 expansion but do not develop the disease. SCA 10 is described in Mexican families and is associated with seizures. SCA 12 is associated with prominent early tremor of the arms and head (of note given this patient's prominent tremor). SCA 17 presents in midlife and the ataxia tends to be associated with cognitive decline and basal ganglia signs (more than the other SCAs).

In patients with a dominant family history, the yield of current genetic testing is still less than 50% in identifying a specific defect. To date, genetic testing for SCA has been normal.

An alternative to SCA would be a mitochondrial disorder. MR spectroscopy of the brain looking for lactate peaks, serum lactate, and pyruvate; mitochondrial DNA studies; and muscle biopsy may provide laboratory evidence in support of a mitochondrial disorder. These studies have been normal in this patient.

■ SELECTED REFERENCES

Di Donato S, Gellera C, Mariotti C. The complex clinical and genetic classification of inherited ataxias. II. Autosomal recessive ataxias. *Neurol Sci* 2001;22:219–228.
Paulson H, Ammache Z. Ataxia and hereditary disorders. *Neurol Clin* 2001;19:759–782.
Subramony SH, Vig PJ, McDaniel DO. Dominantly inherited ataxias. *Semin Neurol* 1999;19:419–425.
The inherited ataxias. In: Conneally M (ed). *Neurogenetics*. Philadelphia Continuum 2000:73–99.

■ SEE QUESTIONS: 27, 85, 143, 241

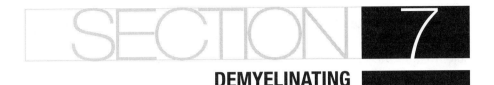

SECTION 7

DEMYELINING

CASE 62

BILATERAL INTERNUCLEAR OPHTHALMOPLEGIA SECONDARY TO MULTIPLE SCLEROSIS

OBJECTIVES

- To briefly discuss multiple sclerosis.
- To discuss internuclear ophthalmoplegia.

VIGNETTE

This 44-year-old woman has a long history of neurological symptoms dating back to the late 1970s. In 1980 she had an acute onset of vertigo, lower extremity weakness, and fatigue. Starting in 1996, the patient began to have an insidious onset of progressive difficulties with urinary incontinence, weakness, and poor balance.

CASE SUMMARY

This 44-year-old woman has had several years of intermittent symptoms, most notably fatigue, dizziness, leg weakness, poor balance, urinary problems, and eye movement difficulties. Her exam is notable for bilateral internuclear ophthalmoplegia, nystagmus, and an ataxic and spastic gait. She has multiple sclerosis (MS).

Multiple sclerosis is a demyelinating disease of the central nervous system that appears to be immune mediated. The clinical diagnosis of MS requires two temporally dissociated attacks of demyelination referable to two geographically separate white matter pathways of the brain or spinal cord. There are several forms of MS described by their course over time including relapsing-remitting, progressive-relapsing, secondary progressive, and primary progressive MS. The most common symptoms at the onset of MS are visual or oculomotor weakness or sensory disturbances and incoordination. The diagnosis is made on clinical grounds with corroboration from objective tests such as brain and spinal cord MRI, spinal fluid analysis, and evoked potentials.

Internuclear ophthalmoplegia (INO) is one of the horizontal disconjugate gaze palsies. The brainstem neurons responsible for conjugate horizontal saccadic eye movements are located in the pons, in particular in the paramedian pontine reticular formation (PPRF) and the interneurons of the abducens nucleus. If one wants to look to the left, the left lateral rectus (abducens nerve) and the right medial rectus (oculomotor nerve) must activate synchronously. The axons of the abducens interneurons cross to the contralateral side in the lower pons and ascend in the medial longitudinal fasciculus (MLF) to the contralateral oculomotor nucleus.

An INO is characterized by adduction weakness of one eye and monocular nystagmus of the abducting eye when one tries to look horizontally in a direction. The adduction weakness results from disruption of the signals carried by the MLF destined for the oculomotor nucleus. A right INO is named for the side of the disrupted MLF (right) and results in poor adduction of the right eye. The pathogenesis of the nystagmus of the abducting eye is unclear. Unilateral or bilateral INOs are most often seen in MS and brainstem infarctions.

■ **SELECTED REFERENCES**

Biller J, ed. *Practical neurology,* 2nd ed. Philadelphia: Lippincott Williams & Wilkins, 2002.
Brazis PW, Masdeu JC, Biller J, eds. *Localization in clinical neurology,* 4th ed. Philadelphia: Lippincott Williams & Wilkins, 2001.

■ **SEE QUESTIONS: 2, 28, 51, 62, 63, 111, 150, 168, 177, 180, 191, 193, 208, 209, 245**

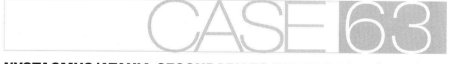

NYSTAGMUS/ATAXIA SECONDARY TO RELAPSING-REMITTING MULTIPLE SCLEROSIS

OBJECTIVES

▓ To discuss relapsing-remitting multiple sclerosis.
▓ To discuss the treatment of MS.

VIGNETTE

A 27-year-old African-American woman had several episodes of neurological deficits. The first episode was characterized by marked fatigue, decreased vision, and unsteadiness. The second episode was characterized by decreased vision in both eyes. The third episode was again characterized by decreased vision and disequilibrium. The latest episode was again associated with decreased vision (20/40 OS, 20/50 OD) and gait unsteadiness.

CASE SUMMARY

This 27-year-old woman has had several episodes of neurologic dysfunction typically involving fatigue, poor vision, and gait unsteadiness. Her examination is notable for nystagmus in nearly all directions of gaze and a cautious and unsteady gait. Her head MRI shows increased T2 signal in her pons, mostly on the left, and bilateral subcortical white matter. She has relapsing-remitting multiple sclerosis (MS).

Multiple sclerosis is a demyelinating disease of the central nervous system that appears to be immune mediated. The clinical diagnosis of MS requires two temporally dissociated attacks of demyelination referable to two geographically separate white matter pathways of the brain or spinal cord. There are several forms of MS, described by their course over time, including relapsing-remitting, progressive-relapsing, secondary progressive, and primary progressive MS. The most common symptoms at the onset of MS are visual or oculomotor weakness or sensory disturbances and incoordination. However, an incredibly wide variety of brain and spinal cord symptoms and signs can occur with MS. The diagnosis is made on clinical grounds with corroboration from objective tests such as brain and spinal cord MRI, spinal fluid analysis, and evoked potentials.

Relapsing-remitting MS is the most common form of MS at presentation. Neurologic dysfunction occurs and may increase over days or weeks, then plateaus, and then resolves over days or weeks. Initially, it is common for patients to recover to normal functioning after these attacks/exacerbations/relapses. MRI of the brain had become one of the most helpful and sensitive tools to help diagnose MS. Images typically reveal multiple focal areas of increased T2 or FLAIR signal in the white matter, particularly the periventricular white matter. If there is a breakdown of the blood–brain barrier, the lesions may demonstrate gadolinium enhancement.

Although there is no cure for MS, the treatment of MS has improved over the years. For acute exacerbations, corticosteroids by mouth or intravenously can be given. The goal of treating relapses is to hasten recovery. A number of immune-modulating therapies have been proven to alter the course of relapsing-remitting over time. These medications decrease the frequency of relapses and often decrease the number of new lesions noted on brain MRI. Interferon β-1a, interferon β-1b, and glatiramer acetate are used in an injectable form. Mitoxantrone, a chemotherapeutic agent, has been shown to be helpful in worsening relapsing-remitting MS but its used is limited by cardiac toxicity.

A number of medications can be used for symptomatic control in patients with MS. A variety of different types of medications can be used to treat such symptoms as spasticity, fatigue, depression, urinary dysfunction, and neurogenic pain.

■ SELECTED REFERENCES

Biller J, ed. *Practical neurology,* 2nd ed. Philadelphia: Lippincott Williams & Wilkins, 2002.
Mattson DH. Alphabet soup: a Personal, evolving, mostly evidence-based and logical, sequential approach to the "ABCNR" drugs in multiple sclerosis. *Semin Neurol* 2002;22(Mar):17–25.

■ SEE QUESTIONS: 28, 51, 111, 150, 168, 177, 180, 191, 193, 208, 209, 245, 257

CASE 64

MULTIPLE SCLEROSIS (PONTINE LESION)

OBJECTIVES

- To discuss the clinical manifestations of a pontine lesion.
- To discuss the tests used to diagnose multiple sclerosis.

VIGNETTE

A 35-year-old man was admitted for evaluation of a subacute onset of right and left hemibody numbness, incoordination, diplopia, and right-sided facial weakness.

CASE SUMMARY

This 35-year-old man was admitted with bilateral numbness, incoordination, diplopia, and right facial weakness. On examination he was noted to have poor abduction of his right eye, nystagmus, and right upper and lower face weakness. He also showed left arm drift and clumsiness, left leg clumsiness, and an ataxic wide-based gait. His head MRI demonstrates hyperintensity in the pons at the level of the middle cerebellar peduncle (much worse on the left) and smaller areas of increased signal in the subcortical white matter of both hemispheres. He has multiple sclerosis (MS).

Although his MRI did show smaller areas of increased signal in the subcortical white matter of both hemispheres, the right pontine lesion appears to be causing most of his symptoms and signs. His poor right eye abduction is due to dysfunction of the abducens nucleus or fascicles in the right pons. However, he does not adduct the left eye well when gazing right. This is suggestive of a right gaze palsy, which would indicate a nuclear right abducens palsy. The abducens nuclear complex coordinates the action of both eyes to a produce horizontal gaze. He demonstrates a "peripheral" right facial weakness in that his frontalis (upper face) and mouth (lower face) movement are equally affected. This is due, however, to a central nervous system lesion of the nucleus or fascicles of the facial nerve.

On attempting to close the eye on the affected side, the eyeball may deviate up and slightly outward. This is called Bell's phenomenon. It is due to relaxation of the inferior rectus and contraction of the superior rectus. It is a normal response that becomes visible because of the weakness of eye closure. However, it may be absent in about 10% of normal people. He also demonstrates a form of ataxic hemiparesis that is often seen with a lesion (commonly an infarct) in the contralateral basis pontis. He has a bit of drift of the arm, but the ataxia noted of the left arm and leg appear more prominent than any weakness. This syndrome has also been associated with dysarthria and nystagmus.

The diagnosis of multiple sclerosis is made on clinical grounds with corroboration from objective tests such as brain and spinal cord MRI, spinal fluid analysis, and evoked potentials. Brain MRI images typically show multiple periventricular areas of increased signal on T2 and FLAIR sequences. Lesions that affect the corpus callosum or that involve white matter of the cerebellum and brainstem are suggestive of MS. Gadolinium-enhancing lesions reflect a breakdown of the blood-brain barrier and usually indicate an active plaque or area of inflammation. Areas of decreased signal on T1 images correlated with areas of brain destruction and have been correlated with disability. Spinal fluid examination may show a pattern suggestive of MS, but these changes are not specific for MS. The opening pressure should be normal. On cell count, a mild lymphocytosis can be seen. The CSF total protein is often mildly elevated.

CSF immunoglobulin levels are typically elevated. The IgG synthesis can be estimated by calculation and may be elevated. The IgG index is a calculation [(CSF IgG/serum IgG)/(CSF albumin/serum albumin)] used to demonstrate an increased amount of IgG present in the CSF compared to serum. It is often greater than 0.7 in patients with MS. Elevated CSF levels of myelin basic protein may be seen in MS. CSF protein electrophoresis frequently demonstrates the presence of oligoclonal bands. Evoked potentials may be helpful if they can demonstrate a lesion not obvious by examination or history that would make the disease process a multifocal one. Visual evoked potentials may show conduction defects in the visual pathways. Somatosensory evoked potentials and brainstem auditory evoked potentials are used to show defects in the somatosensory pathways and auditory pathways, respectively.

■ **SELECTED REFERENCES**

Biller J, ed. *Practical neurology,* 2nd ed. Philadelphia: Lippincott Williams & Wilkins, 2002.

Brazis PW, Masdeu JC, Biller J, eds. *Localization in clinical neurology,* 4th ed. Philadelphia: Lippincott Williams & Wilkins, 2001.

■ **SEE QUESTIONS: 28, 51, 111, 150, 152, 168, 180, 191, 193, 208, 209, 245**

CASE 65

SPASTIC GAIT/DYSARTHRIA DUE TO PRIMARY PROGRESSIVE MULTIPLE SCLEROSIS

OBJECTIVES

▓ To discuss primary progressive multiple sclerosis.
▓ To discuss the treatment of primary progressive multiple sclerosis.

VIGNETTE

This 65-year-old man presents with a 4-year history of left-leg stiffness and weakness. He complains his left foot will "slap" when he walks. A lumbar laminectomy has not improved his symptoms. Recently, his wife has noted he is slurring his speech.

CASE SUMMARY

This 65-year-old man has a 4-year history of progressive lower extremity weakness and stiffness (worse on the left) and more recently noted slurred speech. His exam is notable for increased tone in both legs, a weak left leg, an extensor plantar response on the left, and a spastic gait. He was diagnosed with primary progressive multiple sclerosis (MS).

Multiple sclerosis is a demyelinating disease of the central nervous system that appears to be immune mediated. There are several forms of MS described by their course over time including relapsing-remitting, progressive-relapsing, secondary progressive, and primary progressive MS. Primary progressive MS (PPMS) occurs in about 10% to 15% of patients with MS. It is called primary progressive because of disease progression from the onset although there may be occasional plateaus or temporary minor improvements. The patients do not have the more common and obvious relapses and recoveries. In relapsing-remitting MS (RRMS) there is a preponderance of women over men, but in PPMS the ratio is approximately 1:1.

The most common presentation is a progressive myelopathy, often a spastic paraparesis. MRI changes in the brain and spinal cord, especially gadolinium enhancement, appear less frequently overall in patients with PPMS compared to those with RRMS. PPMS appears to involve less inflammation and more neurodegenerative pathology. PPMS also appears more difficult to treat. None of the currently available immunomodulatory therapies (interferon β-1a, interferon β-1b, glatiramer acetate, mitoxantrone) have been proven to be definitively helpful and have not been approved by the FDA to treat PPMS.

A number of medications can be considered in PPMS including intravenous monthly corticosteroid pulses, methotrexate, cyclophosphamide, cladribine, azothiaprine, and intravenous gamma globulin. Unfortunately, none has been proven to be of significant benefit and most carry the potential for significant side effects. A number of medications can be used for symptomatic control in patients with MS. A variety of different types of medications can be used to treat such symptoms as spasticity, fatigue, depression, urinary dysfunction, and neurogenic pain.

■ SELECTED REFERENCES

Biller J, eds. *Practical neurology,* 2nd ed. Philadelphia: Lippincott Williams & Wilkins, 2002.

Mattson DH. Alphabet soup: a personal, evolving, mostly evidence-based and logical, sequential approach to the "ABCNR" drugs in multiple sclerosis. *Semin Neurol* 2002;22(Mar):17–25.

McDonnell GV, Hawkins SA. Primary progressive multiple sclerosis: increasing clarity but many unanswered questions. *J Neurol Sci* 2002;199:1–15.

■ SEE QUESTIONS: 111, 150, 168, 191, 193, 208, 209, 245

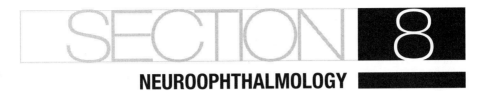

SECTION 8

NEUROOPHTHALMOLOGY

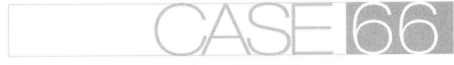

CASE 66

HORNER'S SYNDROME IN PATIENT WITH WALLENBERG SYNDROME

OBJECTIVE

▨ To review the neuroophthalmological manifestations of vertebrobasilar dissections.

VIGNETTE

A 39-year-old woman had a sudden onset of severe left posterior neck pain. She also had left face numbness and left-sided incoordination. She felt veering to the left and vomited on numerous occasions. She had no vertigo, diplopia, dysarthria, tinnitus, hearing loss, or hiccups. She also noted drooping of the left eyelid, and subsequently, she had trouble perceiving heat on the right hemibody and has experienced some dysesthesias of the right leg. The patient had no prior chiropractic manipulations or neck injuries.

CASE SUMMARY

Our patient had a classic history of a lateral medullary syndrome (Wallenberg syndrome) due to a vertebral artery dissection. In addition to her residual dysesthetic sensory symptomatology, she was left with a Horner's syndrome due to her central lesion (i.e., hypothalamospinal pathway at the dorsolateral brainstem tegmentum). A Horner's syndrome results from underactivity of the oculosympathetic pathway, and is characterized by miosis, incomplete eyelid ptosis, and facial anhidrosis. The anisocoria is greater in darkness.

The affected pupil dilates more slowly than the normal pupil (dilation lag). In addition to a first-order neuron Horner's syndrome, other neuroophthalmological manifestations of vertebrobasilar dissections include diplopia, nystagmus, oscillopsia, ocular misalignment, skew deviation, ocular motor nerve palsies (CN III, IV, and VI), lateral gaze palsy, internuclear ophthalmoplegia, and homonymous visual field defects.

■ SELECTED REFERENCES

Love BB, Biller J. Neurovascular system. In: Goetz G, ed. *Textbook of clinical neurology.* Philadelphia: WB Saunders, 2003:395–424.

Love BB, Biller J. Stroke in young adults. In: Samuels MA, Keske SF, eds. *Office practice of neurology,* 2nd ed. New York: Churchill Livingstone, 2003:337–358.

■ SEE QUESTIONS: 59, 113, 114

CASE 67

ADIE'S TONIC PUPIL/ROSS SYNDROME

OBJECTIVES

- To demonstrate a tonic pupil (Adie's tonic pupil).
- To demonstrate testing for light-near dissociation.
- To review pharmacological testing for patients with tonic pupil.
- To review manifestations of Holmes-Adie and Ross syndromes.

VIGNETTE

A 49-year-old man had frequent episodes of heat exhaustion and also noted that he had excessive sweating involving the left lower quadrant of his back associated with lack of sweating in his forehead, axilla, hands, and feet. He also had trouble focusing with his left eye.

CASE SUMMARY

Our patient had episodes of heat exhaustion associated with hyperhidrosis and segmental anhidrosis. He also probably had problems with accommodation of his left eye. Examination was remarkable for anisocoria (left pupil larger than right pupil) with absent reaction to light but a slow constriction to prolonged near effort (light-near dissociation). Redilation after constriction (not shown) was slow and tonic. The patellar and Achilles reflexes were absent.

Our patient had a tonic pupil. Tonic pupils occur due to damage to the ciliary ganglion or the short ciliary nerves, as part of a widespread autonomic neuropathy, or in otherwise healthy individuals (Adie's tonic pupil syndrome). Adie's syndrome may be unilateral or bilateral and may be associated with depressed or absent patellar and Achilles muscle stretch reflexes (Holmes-Adie syndrome). Ross syndrome refers to the clinical condition when a tonic pupil is associated with hyporeflexia and progressive segmental hypohidrosis with compensatory hyperhidrosis.

■ SELECTED REFERENCES

Thompson HS, Miller NR. Disorders of pupillary function, accommodation, and lacrimation. In: Miller NR, Newman NJ, eds. *Walsh and Hoyt's clinical neuro-ophthalmology*, 5th ed. Baltimore: Williams & Wilkins, 1998:1016–1018.

Weller M, Wilhelm H, Sommer N, et al. Tonic pupil, areflexia, and segmental anhidrosis. Two cases of Ross syndrome and review of the literature. *J Neurol* 1992;239:231–234.

■ SEE QUESTIONS: 113, 114, 135

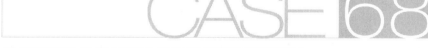

ANTERIOR ISCHEMIC OPTIC NEUROPATHY

OBJECTIVES

■ To name the most common symptom of anterior ischemic optic neuropathy (AION).
■ To name the most common signs and causes of AION.
■ To describe the common visual field abnormalities seen in AION.

VIGNETTE

A 44-year-old woman awoke with a scotoma in the superior visual field of the OD in January 2000. On exam, VA 20/30 OD; 20/20 OS; right optic disc swelling; partial superior altitudinal defect OD. ESR was normal.

CASE SUMMARY

Our patient had painless visual loss of her right eye (OD). She took one tablet of sumatriptan, as she thought she could have a migrainous aura. Her examination was remarkable for decreased visual acuity of the OD, slight edema of the right optic disc, and a relative afferent pupillary defect (RAPD). MRI of the brain and orbits was normal. MRA of the intracranial vessels showed narrowing of the right proximal (A1) segment of the anterior cerebral artery. Catheter arteriogram showed an occluded supraclinoid right internal carotid artery after the origin of the ophthalmic artery. There was also an occluded right P2 segment with a hypoplastic right P1 segment of the posterior cerebral artery (PCA). Further investigations demonstrated normal ESR, CRP, and fasting plasma homocysteine. She was found to be heterozygous for the methylenetetrahydrofolate reductase (MTHFR) gene.

Our patient had optic nerve dysfunction secondary to an ischemic vascular insult. The most common symptom of anterior ischemic optic neuropathy (AION) is acute painless vision loss in one eye. The visual difficulties can range from scotomata to complete monocular visual loss. Examination may reveal poor visual activity in the affected eye, a swollen or edematous optic disc often associated with flame hemorrhages or cotton wool spots around the disc, and a relative afferent pupillary defect (RAPD). Visual field deficits often occur such as altitudinal (especially inferior) defects and central scotoma.

AION is presumably due to occlusion of the posterior ciliary arteries and may be nonarteritic (NA-AION) or arteritic (due to temporal or giant cell arteritis). Carotid artery stenosis is rarely associated with AION. AION may also occur in association with diabetes, migraine, collagen vascular disease, thrombophilic states including the antiphospholipid antibody syndrome, severe arterial hypotension, profound acute blood loss, and after cataract extraction. NA-AION has recently been reported in association with the administration of sildenafil (Viagra). A small cup-to-disc ratio ("a disc at risk") seems to be an additional risk factor for AION.

One must recognize that giant cell arteritis is a cause for arteritic AION as effective therapy in the form of corticosteroids is available. Arteritic AION is often associated with more severe visual loss, and the optic disc swelling tends to have a chalky white appearance. Nonarteritic AION is most commonly caused by atherosclerosis, which is promoted by such risk factors as hypertension and diabetes mellitus. Our patient was diagnosed as having a nonarteritic AION (NA-AION). The patient was treated with aspirin, verapamil, and a combination of folic acid, pyridoxine (vitamin B_6), and cobalamin (vitamin B_{12}) and was told to avoid any sympathomimetic or vasoconstrictive drug. Decompressive surgery for NA-AION is not indicated. In general, prognosis for visual recovery is poor.

■ SELECTED REFERENCES

Brouzas D, Charakidas A, Andrioti E, et al. Non-arteritic anterior ischemic optic neuropathy associated with coexistent factor V Leiden and methylenetetrahydrofolate reductase mutations. *Neuro-Ophthalmology* 2001;26:201–204.

Egan R, Pomeranz H. Sildenafil (Viagra) associated anterior ischemic optic neuropathy. *Arch Ophthalmol* 2000;118:291–292.

Lee AG, Brazis PW. *Clinical pathways in neuro-ophthalmology. An evidence-based approach.* New York: Thieme, 1998.

The Ischemic Optic Neuropathy Decompression Trial Research Group. Optic nerve decompression for non-arteritic ischemic optic neuropathy (NAION) is not effective and may be harmful. *JAMA* 1995;273:625–632.

■ SEE QUESTIONS: 43, 44, 45, 90, 112, 147, 196, 223, 256

CASE 69

POSTOPERATIVE ACUTE LEFT CN III PALSY

OBJECTIVES

▨ To demonstrate the characteristic pattern of a third nerve palsy.
▨ To describe the phenomenology of aberrant regeneration of the third cranial nerve.

VIGNETTE

Following surgery of an intracranial mass lesion, this 60-year-old woman developed a droopy left eyelid and diplopia.

CASE SUMMARY

Our patient had a recent craniotomy for an intracranial mass. On examination, she had a complete left eyelid ptosis. Upon lifting her drooped eyelid, it was noted she had exotropia (lateral deviation) and hypotropia (downward deviation) of the left eye. She also had anisocoria (pupillary asymmetry). The left pupil measured 5 mm in diameter, and the right pupil measured 2 mm in diameter. There was no constriction directly or consensually of the left pupil. She had limited adduction (medial rectus muscle), supraduction (superior rectus and inferior oblique muscles), and infraduction (inferior rectus muscle) of the left eye. On attempted adduction of the left eye, there was normal depression and intorsion (superior oblique muscle). She had full abduction of the left eye (lateral rectus muscle). The range of eye movements was normal on the right eye.

Normal contraction of the medial rectus muscle produces adduction (inward turning), whereas abduction (outward turning) is caused by the lateral rectus muscle. The superior and inferior recti muscles are best evaluated with the eye abducted. Elevation in abduction is caused by the superior rectus muscle. Depression of the globe in abduction is caused by the inferior rectus muscle. The oblique muscles are best evaluated with the eye adducted. Elevation of the eye on adduction is caused by the inferior oblique muscle. Depression of the globe in adduction is caused by the superior oblique.

Why couldn't she open her left eye? With a third nerve lesion, eye opening is impaired. The levator palpebrae superioris, innervated by the third nerve, plays the major role in eye opening. On the other hand, with a cranial nerve VII lesion, eye closure (orbicularis oculi) is impaired, and the palpebral fissure is wider. Why did she have anisocoria? Two iris muscles regulate pupil size. The sphincter (pupilloconstrictor) is innervated by the parasympathetic system, and the dilator (pupillodilator) is innervated by the sympathetic system. As a result of parasympathetic dysfunction, the left pupil became larger and not reactive to light.

In summary, our patient had a left third nerve (CN III) palsy characterized by complete eyelid ptosis, pupillary dilation, impaired pupillary reaction to light, and limitation of adduction, supraduction, and infraduction. The third nerve innervates the levator palpebrae superioris; the superior, inferior, and medial recti; the inferior oblique muscles; and the pupillary constrictors (sphincter pupillae muscle and ciliary muscles). Lesions can affect the third nerve in the midbrain (nucleus or fascicular portion), in the subarachnoid space, in the cavernous sinus, at the superior orbital fissure, or in the orbit.

The oculomotor nuclear complex is located in the midbrain, rostral to the level of the nucleus of cranial nerve IV. The fascicular portion of the third nerve travels ventrally traversing the red nucleus and exits anteriorly medial to the cerebral peduncles. In the subarachnoid space, each third nerve passes between the posterior cerebral and superior cerebellar arteries. The third nerve then enters the lateral wall of the cavernous sinus. The fourth cranial nerve and the first division of the trigeminal nerve (V1) also lie along the lateral wall of the cavernous sinus, whereas the sixth cranial nerve and the oculosympathetic fibers lie more medially. Once it reaches the superior orbital fissure, the third nerve divides into a superior division that innervates the levator palpebrae muscles and the superior rectus and an inferior division that innervates the medial and inferior recti, the inferior oblique, and the presynaptic parasympathetic outflow to the ciliary ganglion.

MRI with gadolinium disclosed a large left cavernous sinus/sphenoid wing mass that proved to be a meningioma. Cranial nerves III, IV, VI, and V1 and sympathetic/parasympathetic connections are present in the cavernous sinus. Blood supply to the cavernous cranial nerves arises from the inferolateral trunk of the internal carotid artery (ICA), and in some cases, from the accessory meningeal artery. Sympathetic fibers extend along the intradural ICA, whereas the parasympathetic fibers and ganglion cells are associated with the cavernous ICA. Lesions affecting the third nerve in the cavernous sinus may be painless or painful. They may occur in isolation or may often compromise cranial nerves four (CN IV), six (CN VI), and the ophthalmic division of cranial nerve five (V1).

Compressive lesions of the third nerve in the cavernous sinus may spare the pupil. Conversely, a third nerve palsy associated with a small pupil (Horner's syndrome) due to oculosympathetic compromise virtually localizes the lesion to the cavernous sinus. Features of primary aberrant regeneration also help localize the lesion to the cavernous sinus and exclude a primary vasculopathic injury such as a diabetic third nerve palsy.

Signs of aberrant regeneration of the third cranial nerve include the following: retraction and elevation of the lid on downward gaze (pseudo-Graefe sign); elevation of the involved lid on attempted adduction of the eye (gaze lid dyskinesis); retraction of the globe on attempted vertical eye movements; adduction of the involved eye on attempted elevation or depression; lack of pupillary reactivity to light, but adequate response when the medial rectus muscle, inferior rectus muscle, or elevators of the eye are activated (pseudo–Argyll Robertson pupil); delayed onset abduction defect; and lagophthalmos.

Aberrant regeneration of the third nerve usually follows injury to the third cranial nerve by intracavernous aneurysms, following aneurysm surgery, or trauma. Aberrant regeneration of the third cranial nerve has also been reported in cases of ophthalmoplegic migraine, a β-lipoproteinemia, and in cases of idiopathic oculomotor nerve palsies.

The differential diagnosis of cavernous sinus lesions also includes intracavernous aneurysms, carotid-cavernous fistulas, pituitary adenoma, pituitary apoplexy, metastases, schwannomas, infections such as mucormycosis or aspergillosis, and idiopathic granulomatous inflammation of the cavernous sinus (Tolosa-Hunt syndrome).

■ SELECTED REFERENCES

Brazis PW, Masdeu JC, Biller J. *Localization in clinical neurology,* 4th ed. Philadelphia: Lippincott Williams & Wilkins, 2001.

Carrasco JR, Savino PJ, Bilyk JR. Primary aberrant oculomotor nerve regeneration from a posterior communicating artery aneurysm. *Arch Ophthalmol* 2002;120:663–665.

Rush JA, Younge BR. Paralysis of cranial nerves III, IV, and VI. *Arch Ophthalmol* 1981;99(Jan):76–79.

Tytle TL, Punukollu PK. Carotid cavernous fistula. In: Biller J ed. *Seminars in cerebrovascular diseases and stroke.* Philadelphia: WB Saunders, 2001;1:83–111.

■ SEE QUESTIONS: 113, 114, 142, 194, 195, 196, 197, 229, 235

CASE 70

PROGRESSIVE LEFT CN III PALSY SECONDARY TO CAVERNOUS SINUS MASS LESION

OBJECTIVES

- To demonstrate the characteristic pattern of a third nerve palsy.
- To discuss differential diagnosis of cavernous sinus mass lesions.

VIGNETTE

A 38-year-old man had a 6-year history of painless progressive left eyelid drooping, trouble with near vision, and horizontal diplopia.

CASE SUMMARY

Our patient had a 6-year history of progressive painless left upper eyelid ptosis and binocular horizontal diplopia, worse on gazing to the right. The patient also had noticed a larger left pupil and had blurred vision with his left eye when looking at near objects.

On examination, visual acuity was 20/20 on the right eye (OD) and 20/25 on the left eye (OS). Confrontation visual fields were normal. On funduscopy, the appearance of the maculae, vessels, and periphery was normal. On center gaze, there was a slight exotropia (lateral deviation) and hypotropia (downward deviation) of the left eye. The range of eye movements was normal on the right eye. There was left upper eyelid ptosis.

He had inability to fully adduct his left eye. With the left eye abducted, he had weakness of elevation and depression of the eye. On attempted adduction of the left eye, there was restricted elevation but normal depression and intorsion. He had full abduction of the left eye. The right pupil measured 2 mm in diameter and the left measured 4 mm. There was no apparent constriction directly or consensually of the left pupil. Corneal sensation was normal. There was no hypesthesia of the left forehead or cheek.

Our patient had a left third nerve (CN III) palsy characterized by eyelid ptosis, pupillary dilation, impaired pupillary reaction to light, and limitation of adduction (medial rectus muscle), supraduction (superior rectus and inferior oblique muscles), and infraduction (inferior rectus muscle). The third nerve innervates the levator palpebrae superioris; the superior, inferior, and medial recti; the inferior oblique muscles; and the pupillary constrictors (sphincter pupillae muscle and ciliary muscles). Lesions can affect the third nerve in the midbrain (nucleus or fascicular portion), in the subarachnoid space, in the cavernous sinus, at the superior orbital fissure, or in the orbit.

MRI with gadolinium disclosed a left cavernous sinus/medial sphenoid wing mass. Lesions affecting the third nerve in the cavernous sinus may be painless or painful. They may occur in isolation or may often compromise cranial nerves four (CN IV), six (CN VI), and the ophthalmic division of cranial nerve V (V1). Compressive lesions of the third nerve in the cavernous sinus may spare the pupil. Conversely, a third nerve palsy associated with a small pupil (Horner's syndrome) due to oculosympathetic compromise virtually localizes the lesion to the cavernous sinus. Features of primary aberrant regeneration also help localize the lesion to the cavernous sinus.

Our patient underwent a left frontotemporal orbitozygomatic craniotomy with subtotal resection of a left cavernous sinus meningioma. Meningiomas account for approximately 15% to 20% of intracranial tumors. Meningiomas are slow-growing tumors and the most common extraaxial tumors in the brain. They arise from arachnoid cells and are more common in women than in men. Most meningiomas are supratentorial. Frequent locations are parasagittal along the falx cerebri and laterally over the cerebral convexity. Other important locations are the olfactory groove, sphenoid wing, juxtasellar region, tentorium, posterior fossa (petrosal), foramen magnus, and clivus. Occasionally, meningiomas are intraventricular. Spinal meningiomas account for approximately 10% of all meningiomas and predominate in the thoracic spine.

Differential diagnosis of cavernous sinus lesions also includes intracavernous aneurysms, carotid-cavernous fistulas, pituitary adenoma, pituitary apoplexy, metastases, schwannomas, infections such as mucormycosis or aspergillosis, and idiopathic granulomatous inflammation of the cavernous sinus (Tolosa-Hunt syndrome). Most patients with ischemic (vasculopathic) third nerve palsies have pupillary sparing and recover within 8 to 12 weeks.

■ **SELECTED REFERENCES**

Ayerbe J, Lobato Rd, de la Cruz J, et al. Risk factors predicting recurrence in patients operated on for intracranial meningioma. A multivariate analysis. *Acta Neurochir (Wien)* 1999;141:921–932.

Biller J, ed. *Practical neurology,* 2nd ed. Philadelphia: Lippincott Williams & Wilkins, 2002.

Brazis PW, Masdeu JC, Biller J. *Localization in clinical neurology,* 4th ed. Philadelphia: Lippincott Williams & Wilkins, 2001.

Rush JA, Younge BR. Paralysis of cranial nerves III, IV, and VI. *Arch Ophthalmol* 1981;99(Jan):76–79.

■ SEE QUESTIONS: 13, 113, 114, 142, 194, 195, 196, 197

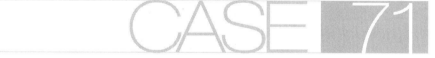

CN VI PALSY

OBJECTIVES

- To describe diagnostic criteria of an abducens (CN VI) palsy.
- To review the topographical locations accounting for abducens (CN VI) palsy.
- To describe potential causes of abducens (CN VI) palsy.

VIGNETTE

An 82-year-old man with a history of hypertension and hyperlipidemia was referred for evaluation of headaches and horizontal diplopia.

CASE SUMMARY

Our patient had a history of arterial hypertension and hyperlipidemia and experienced nonpositional headaches and sudden onset of binocular diplopia with horizontal separation of the images that were worse in the distance. He had no associated scalp or occipital tenderness, eyelid ptosis, or history of thyroid disease. There was no diurnal variation of the diplopia and no fatigability. There was no history of diabetes, sore shoulders or hips, and no jaw claudication. On examination, he had impaired abduction (lateral rectus muscle) of the right eye and nasal deviation (esotropia) of the right eye in center gaze.

There was no proptosis, chemosis, or lid swelling. He had no evidence of eyelid ptosis, papilledema, or a Horner's syndrome. The remainder of his neurological examination was unremarkable. MRI of the brain showed changes compatible with small vessel ischemic disease. There were no brainstem acute ischemic changes on diffusion-weighted MR images. MRA showed minimal tortuosity of the vertebrobasilar system, but no dolichoectasia, aneurysms, or vascular abnormalities. MRI of the orbits was unremarkable.

Our patient had a characteristic history and examination pattern of isolated abducens (CN VI) palsy. There was no evidence of ipsilateral gaze palsy as seen with lesions affecting the abducens nucleus. The abducens nucleus is located in the dorsal lower portion of the pons. The abducens nerve exits the brainstem ventrally at the level of the horizontal sulcus between the pons and medulla and courses anterolaterally passing over the petrous apex to enter the lateral wall of the cavernous sinus. Along with the oculomotor nerve (CN III) and trochlear nerve (CN IV), the abducens nerve enters the orbit through the superior orbital fissure to innervate the lateral rectus muscle.

Movement of the eye nasally is termed adduction; temporal movement is termed abduction. Elevation and depression of the eye are termed supraduction and infraduction, respectively. Intorsion refers to nasal rotation of the 12 o'clock position on the vertical meridian; extorsion is temporal rotation of the 12 o'clock position on the vertical meridian. The abducens nerve supplies the lateral rectus muscle. The lateral rectus muscle has only horizontal actions and is the primary abductor of the eye.

A sixth nerve palsy may be the result of nuclear, fascicular, subarachnoid, cavernous, or orbital lesions. Etiologies of sixth nerve palsies are myriad including ischemic and hemorrhagic disorders; aneurysms or other vascular anomalies; demyelinating, neoplastic, metabolic, traumatic, inflammatory/infectious disorders; hydrocephalus; raised intracranial pressure; or CSF hypotension. However, despite extensive investigations, the etiology of a sixth nerve palsy remains undetermined in a considerable number of adults and children.

As in our patient, the most common etiologic factor of a sixth nerve palsy in older adults is microvascular occlusion of the abducens nerve, also known as a vasculopathic sixth nerve palsy. Most vasculopathic sixth nerve palsies recover over a period of 3 to 6 months. Isolated sixth nerve palsies have also been described due to pontine strokes. Our patient had a complete resolution of symptoms in 3 months.

■ **SELECTED REFERENCES**

Biller J, ed. *Practical neurology,* 2nd ed. Philadelphia: Lippincott Williams & Wilkins, 2002.

Brazis PW, Masdeu JC, Biller J. *Localization in clinical neurology* 4th ed. Philadelphia: Lippincott Williams & Wilkins, 2001.

Fukutake T, Hirayama K. Isolated abducens nerve palsy from pontine infarction in a diabetic patient. *Neurology* 1992;42:226.

Rush JA, Younge BR. Paralysis of cranial nerves III, IV, and VI. *Arch Ophthalmol* 1981;99(Jan):76–79.

■ **SEE QUESTIONS: 215, 235**

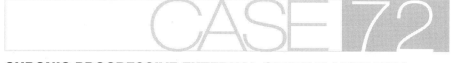

CHRONIC PROGRESSIVE EXTERNAL OPHTHALMOPLEGIA

OBJECTIVES

▥ To discuss the clinical features of chronic progressive external ophthalmoplegia (CPEO).
▥ To review modes of inheritance of CPEO.
▥ To discuss the differential diagnosis with myasthenia gravis.

VIGNETTE

At the age of 23, this 48-year-old woman developed diplopia. Thereafter, she described a history of sudden stepwise impairment of eye movements in both eyes. On exam, VA was 20/30 OD, and pinhole increased acuity to 20/20; 20/100 OS, and pinhole increased acuity to 20/40. Visual fields were full. The fundus was normal and there was no pigmentary retinopathy. The pupils were 4 mm and 4.5 mm in diameter with normal reaction and no RAPD. Ocular motility is shown.

CASE SUMMARY

At the age of 23, our patient suddenly developed diplopia with a defect in abduction of the right eye. This was preceded by a 2-week history of a sharp needlelike pain behind that eye. Thereafter, she described a history of sudden stepwise impairment of eye movements in both eyes. In 1994, she developed severe ptosis of the left upper lid. Because of severe ophthalmoplegia of the right eye and tonic deviation downward of that eye, she had strabismus surgery to elevate the globe. She continued to have intermittent headaches.

Subsequently, she had some bowel incontinence and also complained of occasional dizziness, which was probably related to head movements and the severe limitation of her eye movements. She also had occasional dull aching bitemporal headaches throughout the day and had more difficulty seeing at night. She had no skeletal muscle weakness, hearing loss, seizures, cerebella ataxia, or history of diabetes or other endocrinopathy. She had no variability of her left lid ptosis and did not complain of dryness of her eyes.

On examination, she was of normal stature and was a well-appearing middle-aged woman, except for a slight chin-up head position and a complete ptosis of the left upper lid. There was no sign of exophthalmos. Visual acuity was 20/30-1 in the right eye; pinhole increased acuity to 20/20. Visual acuity in the left eye was 20/100 without correction; pinhole increased acuity to 20/40. Confrontation visual fields were full. On color vision examination, she identified 11 out of 15 plates with each eye. Ocular motility showed that both eyes were tonically deviated slightly in downgaze.

In the right eye, the visual axis was in about 5 degrees of downward gaze. She could move the eye further down by an additional 10 degrees. There were only a few degrees of horizontal movement. In the left eye, the visual axis was almost in center gaze. There were an additional 10 degrees of infraduction in that eye. No horizontal movements were seen. The very small amplitude residual saccades in both eyes horizontally and vertically were extremely slow. No quiver eye movements were seen. Oculocephalic and Bell's eye movements were absent.

The right pupil was 4 mm in diameter, and the left pupil was 4.5 mm in diameter. Their reactions were normal and there was no relative afferent pupillary defect. There was complete ptosis of the left upper lid. Funduscopy showed normal appearance of the discs, vessels, and periphery. There was a slight accentuation of the pigmentation pattern in the macula, but no definite sign of pigmentary retinopathy. The remainder of the neurological examination was unremarkable.

Our patient had extensive evaluations, including unremarkable MRI scans of the orbits and brain, CSF analyses, edrophonium (Tensilon) tests, thyroid function tests, and blood tests for mitochondrial disorders. Serum lactic acid and pyruvic acid were normal. An electroretinogram was performed for photopic and scotopic reactions; the results were normal. Repetitive stimulation studies and single-fiber EMG were unremarkable in many occasions. Chest CT was normal. Biopsy of the left vastus lateralis muscle showed moderate perifascicular atrophy, mild angulated muscle fibers, and increased fat in the muscle fibers, findings that were not conclusive. Southern blot analysis of the skeletal muscle mitochondrial DNA was normal.

She also had a biopsy of two of her extraocular muscles that were fibrotic in nature. Acetylcholine receptor antibodies, except for only one occasion that yielded a positive result, were not detectable. Antistriational (skeletal) antibodies and anti-MuSK antibodies were not detectable. EKG did not show any conduction abnormality. Trials of coenzyme Q (CoQ10), vitamin E, menadione (vitamin K_3), riboflavin, carnitine, corticosteroids, cholinesterase inhibitors (mestinon), mycophenylate mofetil, and intravenous immunoglobulin therapy were unsuccessful.

Our patient probably had an unusual presentation of chronic progressive external ophthalmoplegia (CPEO). CPEO encompasses different conditions characterized by slowly progressive paralysis of the external ocular muscles combined with ptosis. Patients typically have bilateral and symmetrical ophthalmoparesis and ptosis. The ciliary and iris muscles are not involved. Due to the symmetric restriction of eye movements, unlike myasthenia gravis, patients seldom complain of diplopia. Cases have been described with ophthalmoplegia but no ptosis, or with unilateral or asymmetric ptosis.

CPEO may occur in isolation or may be associated with a constellation of ophthalmologic, neurologic, or systemic features. If the ophthalmoplegia appears before age 20, is accompanied by atypical retinitis pigmentosa (salt and pepper pattern), along with a cerebellar ataxia, cardiac conduction defects, and elevated CSF protein (greater than 100 mg/dL), the condition is known as Kearns-Sayre Syndrome (KSS). Other abnormalities in KSS may include short stature, hearing loss, vestibular dysfunction, pendular nystagmus, Babinski sign, delayed puberty, and various other endocrine disorders.

The extraocular muscles are primarily involved in many mitochondrial diseases. CPEO is considered the most frequent form of mitochondrial encephalomyopathies. In addition to the preferential involvement of the ocular and cranial musculature, mitochondrial encephalomyopathies are often associated with dysfunction in other organ systems. Some mitochondrial disorders are associated with prominent vascular headaches. Mitochondrial encephalomyopathies are a complex group of disorders arising from mtDNA mutations. Most cases occur sporadically.

Familial cases have been described. Modes of inheritance include maternal transmission associated with mitochondrial point mutations, autosomal recessive inheritance, and autosomal dominant inheritance. Differentiation of CPEO from other neurogenic, neuromuscular junction or myogenic disorders may be difficult. In the case of our patient, the extreme asymmetry characterizing the onset of the ophthalmoplegia and seen in the lid ptosis of the left were unusual. The history of stepwise progressive loss of eye movements and the presence of diplopia were unusual as well.

However, by history, the careful evaluation for other causes of ophthalmoplegia had been negative. A major concern with an atypical presentation of myasthenia gravis motivated the therapeutic trials of mestinon, corticosteroids, mycophenylate mofetil, and intravenous immunoglobulins. Her greater difficulty with vision at night was probably related to impaired ability to use visual clues for orientation and balance. She did notice dizziness on rapid eye movements of the head, which was probably due to the absence of effective vestibular ocular movements.

■ SELECTED REFERENCES

DiMauro S, Hirano M, Schon EA. Mitochondrial encephalomyopathies: therapeutic approaches. *Neurol Sci* 2000;21:S901–S908.

Lee AG, Brazis PW. Chronic progressive external ophthalmoplegia. *Curr Neurol Neurosci Rep* 2002;2:413–417.

Sahashi K, Yoneda M, Ohno K, et al. Functional characterisation of mitochondrial tRNA (Tyr) mutation (5877—>GA) associated with familial chronic progressive external ophthalmoplegia. *J Med Genet* 2001;38:703–705.

Shrama NK, Gujrati M, Kumar J, et al. Chronic asymmetric progressive external ophthalmoplegia with right facial weakness: a unique presentation of mitochondrial myopathy. *J Neurol Neurosurg Psychiatry* 2002;73(1):95.

■ **SEE QUESTIONS: 2, 231**

CASE 73

RIGHT HOMONYMOUS HEMIANOPIA, ANTIPHOSPHOLIPID ANTIBODY (PCA OCCLUSION)

OBJECTIVES

▒ To review the neuroophthalmological manifestations of posterior cerebral artery (PCA) territory infarcts.
▒ To discuss the differential diagnosis of PCA infarcts in patients with a history of migraines.
▒ To summarize the main neurological manifestations associated with the antiphospholipid antibody syndrome (APAS).
▒ To caution against the premature diagnosis of migrainous cerebral infarction.

VIGNETTE

A 34-year-old woman with a history of migraine headaches had a sudden onset of loss of peripheral vision of the right side of her visual fields. She also had a brief episode of horizontal diplopia and bifrontal headache. She had no nausea, vomiting, or photo- or phonophobia.

CASE SUMMARY

Our patient had an isolated congruous right homonymous hemianopia respecting the vertical meridian due to an occlusion of cortical branches of the left posterior cerebral artery (PCA). A unilateral PCA infarction may produce a contralateral homonymous hemianopia with macular sparing rather than macular splitting. MRA of the extracranial vertebral arteries was unremarkable. There was an occluded P2CA segment with lack of visualization of the calcarine artery, parietooccipital artery, and posterior temporal artery on the intracranial MRA.

Further investigations failed to demonstrate a cardiac source of embolism. As shown by the MRA, she had no evidence of a more proximal vertebrobasilar source, nor evidence of intrinsic atheromatous disease of the PCA system. She did not smoke cigarettes, nor was she on oral contraceptives. Although our patient had a history of migraine headaches, and cerebral infarctions complicating migraine mostly involve the distribution of the PCA, she was found to have persistent elevations of antiphospholipid antibodies titer. Her infarction was attributed to a prothrombotic state due to a primary antiphospholipid antibody syndrome (APAS).

The PCAs arise from the termination of the basilar artery in most patients. Occasionally, one or rarely both PCAs arise from the internal carotid artery from a large posterior communicating artery. The PCAs and their branches supply the mamillary bodies, the thalami, and the medial and basal temporal lobes, including the hippocampi. The manifestations with PCA territory infarctions are variable, depending on the site of occlusion and the availability of collateral blood flow. Occlusion of the precommunal P1 segment causes midbrain, thalamic, and hemispheric infarction.

Occlusion of the PCA in the proximal ambient segment before branching in the thalamogeniculate pedicle causes lateral thalamic and hemispheral symptoms. Occlusions also may affect a single PCA branch, primarily the calcarine artery, or cause a large hemispheric infarction of the PCA territory. Unilateral infarctions in the distribution of the hemispheral branches of the PCA may produce a contralateral homonymous hemianopia caused by infarction of the striate cortex, the optic radiations, or the lateral geniculate body.

There is partial or complete macular sparing if the infarction does not reach the occipital pole. The visual field may be limited to a quadrantanopia. A superior quadrantanopia is caused by infarction of the striate cortex inferior to the calcarine fissure or the inferior optic radiations in the temporooccipital lobes. An inferior quadrantanopia is the result of an infarction of the striate cortex superior to the calcarine fissure or the superior optic radiations in the parietooccipital lobes. Patients with unilateral homonymous hemianopias due to occipital lobe lesions have a normal optokinetic response.

More complex visual changes may also occur with PCA territory infarctions, including formed or unformed visual hallucinations, visual and color agnosias, or prosopagnosia. The syndrome of alexia without agraphia is shown in case 23.

APAS may be primary or secondary to underlying diseases such as systemic lupus erythematosus (SLE), rheumatoid arthritis, Sjögren's syndrome, Sneddon syndrome (livedo reticularis and ischemic cerebrovascular disease), malignancies, syphilis, acute and chronic infections including AIDS, inflammatory bowel disease; administration of certain drugs; liver transplantation; early onset severe preeclampsia; and also in individuals without demonstrable underlying disorder. Ischemic stroke is the most common arterial thrombotic event in APAS.

Reported neurologic involvement associated with antiphospholipid antibodies includes ischemic strokes, TIAs, ocular ischemia, migrainous-like events, cerebral venous thrombosis, dementia (with or without Snedddon syndrome), acute ischemic encephalopathy, transient global amnesia, seizures, chorea, transverse myelopathy, and Guillain-Barré syndrome. Oral anticoagulation with warfarin is the preferred treatment for the prevention of thromboembolic events in patients with APAS.

Warfarin should be replaced by low molecular weight heparin or unfractionated heparin in case of pregnancy.

The use of antiplatelet drugs is also reasonable in the prevention of thrombosis in APAS if anticoagulation is contraindicated. Antimalarial drugs might be useful in APAS patients with or without associated SLE. Our patient received warfarin. Migrainous infarction is a rare event, considering the high prevalence of migraine in the general population. Migraine may increase the risk of ischemic stroke in young women, especially if they also have other risk factors such as smoking and use of oral contraceptives.

■ SELECTED REFERENCES

Caplan LR. *Posterior circulation disease. Clinical findings, diagnosis, and management.* Boston: Blackwell Science, 1996.

Cuadrado MJ, Hughes GRV. Antiphospholipid (Hughes) syndrome. *Rheum Dis Clin North Am* 2001;27:507–524.

Levine SR, Welch KMA. The spectrum of neurologic disease associated with antiphospholipid antibodies. Lupus anticoagulants and anticardiolipin antibodies. *Arch Neurol* 1987;44:876–883.

Tzourio C, Tehindrazanarivelo A, Iglesias S, et al. Case-control study of migraine and risk of ischemic stroke in young women. *Br Med J* 1995;310:830–833.

■ SEE QUESTIONS: 29, 47, 48, 52, 54, 90, 147, 167, 223

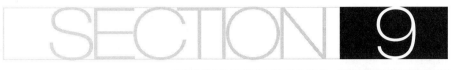

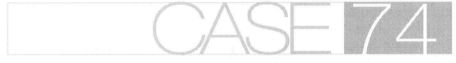

CASE 74

HERPES ZOSTER (POSTHERPETIC NEURALGIA)

OBJECTIVES

- To review the most frequent neurological complications associated with VZV infections.
- To review the clinical presentation and management of uncomplicated herpes zoster.

VIGNETTE

A 63-year-old man had left-sided chest pain and a skin rash.

CASE SUMMARY

Following initial infection, usually as varicella (chickenpox) in childhood, VZV, a DNA virus, remains dormant in the dorsal spinal root ganglion neurons and the fifth cranial nerve (CN V) ganglion neurons. Upon reactivation, a spectrum of clinical manifestations may occur including herpes zoster (shingles), postherpetic neuralgia, cranial neuropathies, Ramsay-Hunt syndrome (geniculate neuralgia, nervus intermedius neuralgia, or herpes zoster oticus), myelitis, radiculitis, brachial plexus neuritis, motor neuropathies, encephalitis, thrombotic cerebral vasculopathy, keratitis, and so forth. Once VZV infection resolves, many patients continue to suffer from pain (postherpetic neuralgia).

Our patient had a typical painful dermatomal rash associated with reactivation of VZV infection. The gradual onset of unilateral dermatomal paresthesias may precede the onset of pain. Dermatomal pain is the most common symptom of zoster and may antedate the cutaneous eruption by days to weeks. After a prodromal illness, erythematous macules and papules appear and progress to vesicles. They then begin to crust and resolve. The crusts usually resolve within 2 to 3 weeks. Patients may experience pain and sensory loss in the distribution of the rash.

Motor weakness, especially in cervical and lumbar radicular distributions, may be overlooked. Zoster typically affects a single dermatome, most commonly a thoracic dermatome. The dermatomes most commonly involved are T5 and T6. However, multiple contiguous or noncontiguous dermatomes may be involved. The ophthalmic division of the fifth cranial nerve (CN V) is the most frequently affected cranial nerve. Rarely, VZV reactivation can occur without cutaneous vesicles (zoster sine herpete).

For typical zoster in an immunocompetent patient, nonopioid analgesics and local anesthetic creams have been used. Whether treatment with oral antiviral agents is essential for typical (noncephalic) herpes zoster is a matter for debate. Immunosuppression increases the risk of VZV infections.

■ **SELECTED REFERENCES**

Kost RG, Starus SE. Postherpetic neuralgia-pathogenesis, treatment, and prevention. *N Engl J Med* 1996; 335:32–42.

Mahalingam R, Wellish MC, Dueland AN, et al. Localization of herpes simplex virus and varicella zoster virus DNA in human ganglia. *Ann Neurol* 1992;31:444–448.

■ **SEE QUESTIONS: 157, 158, 165**

CASE **75**

RECURRENT ASEPTIC MENINGITIS

OBJECTIVES

▓ To define aseptic meningitis.
▓ To name the common causes of aseptic meningitis.
▓ To discuss Mollaret's meningitis.

VIGNETTE

A 34-year-old African-American woman was admitted with new-onset bilateral frontal headaches; posterior neck pain; vomiting; photophobia; numbness in face, arms, and legs; and generalized weakness. She had no fever and denied ill contacts, recent foreign travel, skin lesions, or upper respiratory symptoms. On examination, blood pressure was 137/74 mmHg, heart rate was 92 beats/min, respirations were 18 breaths/min, and temperature was 97.1°F.

CASE SUMMARY

Our patient had three recurrent episodes of headaches, posterior neck pain and stiffness, nausea, vomiting, and fever. Examination showed neck stiffness manifested by limited flexion of the neck on AP direction. She did not have a Brudzinski sign (the patient did not exhibit flexion of her knees and hips when passive flexion of her neck was attempted in the supine position). CSF studies (1999, 2000, 2002) demonstrated a discrete lymphocytic pleocytosis with normal glucose, minimal elevation of protein content, and negative Gram stain, a profile compatible with the diagnosis of aseptic meningitis (Table 75.1). We concluded that our patient had three episodes of recurrent self-limited aseptic meningitis, probably representing a case of Mollaret's meningitis.

Aseptic meningitis is a diagnosis given to patients with clinical and laboratory evidence of meningeal inflammation with negative routine bacterial cultures. The clinical presentation often includes headache (100%), fever (93%), neck stiffness, nausea, vomiting, and confusion. Signs of meningeal irritation include Brudzinski sign (noted previously) and Kernig sign. A positive Kernig sign is present when extension of the knee in a patient lying supine with the hips flexed 90 degrees elicits pain or resistance in the lower back or posterior thigh. CSF generally demonstrates lymphomonocytic pleocytosis (fewer than 500 cells), moderately elevated protein, and normal glucose and lactate levels.

The term *aseptic meningitis* is often used to describe a viral meningitis, but there are multiple infectious and noninfectious causes. Infectious conditions may be viral or nonviral. Viral disorders causing aseptic meningitis syndrome include the following: enterovirus, herpes simplex virus (HSV) 1 and 2, varicella-zoster virus, adenovirus, Epstein-Barr virus, lymphocytic choriomeningitis virus, human immunodeficiency virus, arbovirus, and influenza virus Types A and B. Enteroviruses are the most common cause of viral aseptic meningitis. Bacterial disorders causing aseptic meningitis syndrome include the following: partially treated bacterial meningitis, parameningeal infections, infective endocarditis, *M. pneumoniae, M. tuberculosis,* Ehrlichiosis, *B. burgdorferi, T. pallidum, Brucella* sp., and *Leptospira* sp.

Fungal disorders causing aseptic meninigitis syndrome include *C. neoformans, H. capsulatum, C. immitis,* and *B. dermatitidis.* Parasitic disorders causing the aseptic meningitis syndrome include *T. gondii* and *T. solium.*

Noninfectious causes of the aseptic meningitis syndrome include certain drugs and systemic diseases. Most drug-induced cases are due to nonsteroidal antiinflammatory drugs, antimicrobials, intravenous immunoglobulins, intrathecal agents, and vaccinations. Nonsteroidal antiinflammatory drugs probably account for most of the drug-related cases. Systemic diseases causing the aseptic meningitis syndrome include the following: sarcoidosis, systemic lupus erythematosus, Wegener's granulomatosis, CNS vasculitis, Behçet disease, Vogt-Koyanagi and Harada syndromes, leptomeningeal cancer, posttransplantation lymphoproliferative disorder, and others.

TABLE 75.1: RECURRENT ASEPTIC MENINGITIS

Year	CSF WBC (% lymphocytes)	CSF RBC	CSF Protein	CSF Glucose (serum glucose)
1999	15 (99%)	3	69	52
2000	501 (97%)	72	Not recorded	Not recorded
2002	160 (97%)	4	54	54 (90)

CSF, cerebrospinal fluid; WBC, white blood count; RBC, red blood count.

Mollaret's meningitis is a condition where recurrent episodes of fever are associated with an aseptic meningitis syndrome. The episodes are typically self-limited. No definitive cause has been noted although HSV-2, and less frequently HSV-1, is thought to be the etiology in many cases. This would make acyclovir a reasonable treatment option in patients with Mollaret's meningitis.

■ SELECTED REFERENCES

Jolles S, Sewell WA, Leighton C. Drug-induced aseptic meningitis: diagnosis and management. *Drug Saf* 2000;22(Mar):215–226.

Nowak DA, Boehmer R, Fuchs HH. A retrospective clinical, laboratory and outcome analysis in 43 cases of acute aseptic meningitis. *Eur J Neurol* 2003;10(May):271–280.

Roos K. Viral meningitis and aseptic meningitis. In: Roos K, ed. *Central nervous system infectious diseases and therapy.* New York: Marcel Dekker Inc, 1997:127–139.

■ SEE QUESTIONS: 137, 151, 153, 154, 155, 163, 165

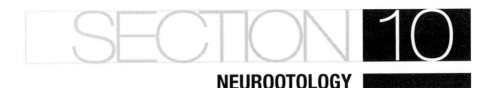

SECTION 10

NEUROOTOLOGY

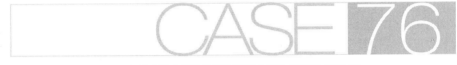

CASE 76

VERTIGO/IMBALANCE SECONDARY TO ISOLATED VERMIAN INFARCTION

OBJECTIVES

- To highlight pitfalls in the diagnosis of acute isolated severe vertigo.
- To review the clinical presentation of the acute vestibular syndrome.
- To describe vascular and nonvascular causes of the central vestibular syndrome.

VIGNETTE

A 62-year-old man experienced a sudden onset of dizziness, vertigo, imbalance, and blurred vision after suddenly turning his head to the right. This was followed by nausea and diaphoresis. The episode lasted for 12 hours.

CASE SUMMARY

Our patient had an attack of acute onset of vertigo and imbalance on suddenly turning his head to the right lasting 12 hours. He had some nausea and diaphoresis. There were no symptoms of upper respiratory infection or flulike illness prior to the onset of vertigo, and he did not complain of auricular pain, hearing loss, tinnitus, aural fullness, emesis, headaches, diplopia, dysarthria, facial paresthesias, extremity weakness, clumsiness, or numbness. He had no sense of being pushed down or to one side (pulsion) and did not have orthostatic hypotension or evidence of a vesicular rash in the external auditory canal and concha. He had no history of motion intolerance during car, boat, or air travel. He was initially misdiagnosed as having presyncope versus syncope, and extensive cardiac investigations were initiated that were unremarkable.

Balance involves the overlapping function of the visual, proprioceptive, and vestibular systems. Vertigo is defined as an illusion of movement either of the self or the environment. Our patient had an acute vestibular syndrome characterized by severe vertigo, nausea, and postural instability. As Neurology was not consulted at the time of presentation, we cannot comment as to the presence of spontaneous nystagmus. When an acute vestibular syndrome evolves over days in an otherwise healthy patient, it is often attributed to a viral vestibular neuritis (vestibular neuronitis). If there is associated hearing loss, it is often attributed to a neurolabyrinthitis.

Vestibular neuritis refers to a disorder of the vestibular system without associated hearing loss, characterized by sudden attacks of severe vertigo, nausea, vomiting, and abnormal vestibular function on caloric testing in otherwise healthy patients. An upper respiratory infection often precedes this condition. The vertigo usually resolves within a week. Viral labyrinthitis is characterized by the acute onset of severe and often incapacitating vertigo, frequently associated with nausea and vomiting. Hearing loss is also present. The vertigo usually resolves over several days to weeks. Bacterial labyrinthitis is rare in the postantibiotic era.

Benign paroxysmal positional vertigo (BPPV), probably the most common cause of vertigo, is characterized by sudden vertigo lasting less than 1 minute that occurs when trying to sit up suddenly, rolling over in bed, or tilting the head backward. Classic BBPV involves the posterior semicircular canal. Cervical vertigo (a controversial entity) is associated with head extension and attributed to vascular compression of the vertebral arteries. As shown by the MRI studies, our patient had central vertigo due to a small caudal vermian infarction.

Vascular causes of the central vestibular syndrome include vertebrobasilar transient ischemic attacks, labyrinthine stroke, Wallenberg syndrome, migraine-associated vertigo, basilar artery migraine (Bickerstaff), subclavian steal syndrome, and cerebellar infarction and hemorrhage. Nonvascular causes of central vertigo include cerebellar, brainstem, and temporal lobe tumors; CNS infections; multiple sclerosis; Chiari malformation; Wernicke's encephalopathy; trauma; focal seizures; and familial periodic ataxia syndromes.

Emergency room physicians should have a low threshold for obtaining consultation with a neurologist or neurosurgeon in patients who present with isolated vertigo or with vertigo, imbalance, and nausea and who also have risk factors for cerebrovascular disease. As many as 25% of patients with cerebrovascular risk factors who present to an emergency room with isolated vertigo, nystagmus, and postural instability have an infarction involving the inferior cerebellum.

■ **SELECTED REFERENCES**

Brazis PW, Masdeu JC, Biller J. *Localization in clinical neurology,* 4th ed. Philadelphia: Lippincott Williams & Wilkins, 2001.

Hotson JR, Baloh RW. Acute vestibular syndrome. *New Engl J Med* 1998;339:680–685.

Norrving B, Magnusson M, Holtas S. Isolated acute vertigo in the elderly: vestibular or vascular disease? *Acta Neurol Scand* 1995;91:43–48.

■ **SEE QUESTIONS: 19, 64, 65, 143**

CASE 77

DEAFNESS/TINNITUS SECONDARY TO VESTIBULAR (ACOUSTIC) SCHWANNOMA

OBJECTIVES

■ To review the importance of a detailed evaluation of tinnitus and hearing loss.
■ To discuss the different clinical manifestations of vestibular schwannomas.
■ To illustrate other etiologies of the cerebellopontine angle syndrome.
■ To analyze potential management strategies for vestibular schwannomas.

VIGNETTE

A 57-year-old man was evaluated because of a 3- to 4-month history of progressive unilateral hearing loss and tinnitus of the right ear.

CASE SUMMARY

Our patient had progressive unilateral sensorineural hearing loss and subjective (audible only to the affected) nonpulsatile tinnitus. MRI of the internal auditory canals demonstrated a small enhancing mass consistent with a small right vestibular schwannoma. Vestibular schwannomas arise in the internal auditory canal in the cerebellopontine angle. Commonly but improperly called "acoustic neuromas," these tumors originate from the vestibular Schwann cells of CN VIII (cochleovestibular nerve) in the internal auditory canal at the glial–Schwann cell junction.

The lesion arises from the inferior or superior division of the vestibular nerve, but it typically causes symptoms due to mass effect on the adjacent cochlear nerve. In the internal auditory canal, the vestibular division of the cochleovestibular nerve courses in the posterior superior and inferior quadrants, and the cochlear division courses in the inferior-posterior quadrant. Besides vestibular schwannomas, other conditions causing the cerebellopontine angle syndrome include meningiomas, lipomas, cholesteatomas, arachnoid cysts, epidermoids, hemangiomas, vascular loops, vertebral dolichoectasia, arteriovenous malformations, and metastatic tumors.

Vestibular schwannomas are slow-growing benign tumors, accounting for approximately 10% of all intracranial tumors. Vestibular schwannomas are the most common cranial nerve schwannomas, followed by schwannomas of the trigeminal and facial nerves. Patients with vestibular schwannomas typically present with insidious cochlear nerve dysfunction, characterized by unilateral high-pitched tinnitus and progressive sensorineural hearing loss with early loss of speech discrimination. Rarely deafness may occur suddenly, most likely due to intratumoral hemorrhage or disruption of regional blood flow due to internal auditory artery occlusion.

A sense of imbalance or disequilibrium is a more frequent complaint than vertigo. As the tumor grows, the internal auditory meatus progressively widens and complete ipsilateral deafness ensues. With medial tumor growth, neighboring cranial nerves are affected, and eventually brainstem and cerebellar compromise occurs with very large tumors. Progressive tumoral enlargement may account for symptoms related to hydrocephalus or symptoms of increased intracranial pressure.

Dysfunction of neighboring cranial nerves varies according to the direction of tumoral growth. With anterior extension, the trigeminal nerve (CN V) and abducens nerve (CN VI) are compromised. With posteroinferior tumoral extension, the glossopharyngeal (CN IX), vagus (CN X), and spinal accessory (CN XI) may be involved. In either case, the facial nerve (CN VII) is usually involved. In patients presenting with bilateral vestibular schwannomas, neurofibromatosis type 2 should be suspected. MRI with gadolinium enhancement is the preferred imaging modality to detect vestibular schwannomas. Vestibular schwannomas often demonstrate enhancement with gadolinium. Pure tone and speech audiometry should be obtained. Brainstem auditory evoked responses are abnormal in the majority of patients.

Management strategies include observation, surgery, and radiation therapy. Cerebellopontine angle mass lesions are usually surgically removed on an elective basis. The goal of surgery is to remove the tumor and preserve facial nerve function. Our patient was treated with stereotactic radiosurgery (gamma knife radiosurgery). Lesions smaller than 3 cm, particularly when there is no brainstem compression or in poor surgical risk patients, are often treated with stereotactic radiosurgery.

■ **SELECTED REFERENCES**

Biller J, ed. *Practical neurology*, 2nd ed. Philadelphia: Lippincott Williams & Wilkins, 2002.

Brazis PW, Masdeu JC, Biller J. *Localization in clinical neurology*, Philadelphia: Lippincott Williams & Wilkins, 2001.

Hart RG, Davenport J. Diagnosis of acoustic neuroma. *Neurosurgery* 1991;9:450–463.

■ **SEE QUESTIONS: 38, 63, 64, 65, 166, 176, 197**

CASE 78

VERTIGINOUS DIZZINESS

OBJECTIVES

▒ To review classification of the common causes of dizziness.
▒ To outline the differential diagnosis of vertigo.

▨ To summarize management of Ménière's disease and benign positional vertigo.

VIGNETTE

A 44-year-old man had recurrent feelings of dizziness and subjective sensations of profound environmental spin. He had occasional off and on high-pitched ringing in both ears, but never simultaneously. Past medical history was noteworthy for deep vein thrombosis of the lower extremity 11 years ago following a fracture. Neurological and neurootologic examinations were normal.

CASE SUMMARY

The patient is a 45-year-old man who presents with a 1-year history of intermittent vertiginous dizziness. He has no hearing loss or fullness, but describes an occasional high-pitched ringing in both ears. MRI scan of the brain with and without contrast and additional extensive laboratory evaluation reveal no etiology for his vertigo.

The four primary categories of dizziness are vertigo, presyncopal dizziness (impending faint), disequilibrium (poor balance), and a nonspecific group. Vertigo is an illusion of spinning or motion, can be any direction, and ranges from mild to intense. Otologic or peripheral vertigo may be present with pathology in the labyrinth or in the vestibular nerve, characterized by intense episodic vertigo, often leaving the patient immobile from the attack of motion sickness. There is often nausea, vomiting, tachycardia, diaphoresis, and severe dysphoria. In contrast, patients with presyncopal dizziness experience light-headedness, feeling as if they might pass out. Causes of presyncopal dizziness include orthostatic hypotension, autonomic neuropathy, antihypertensive medications, vasovagal attacks, and cardiac rhythm problems.

Patients with the third category of dizziness, disequilibrium, use such descriptions as their "balance is off" or they have a "floating feeling." Causes include medication effects, brainstem or cerebellar dysfunction, deafferentation from cervical spondylosis or sensory neuropathy, and degenerative conditions such as parkinsonism. The fourth group of patients with dizziness includes those who do not conform to the other three categories, and such patients often describe vague nonspecific symptoms or have multiple somatic complaints.

Ménière's disease is characterized by recurrent episodes of intense vertigo, tinnitus, hearing loss, and fullness in the head or ears. The condition may be related to prior trauma, infection, or hereditary factors, and in many cases there is no clear trigger. The diagnosis is based on the collection of symptoms. Ménière's disease tends to be recurrent and increases with age; it is related to an accumulation of fluid/endolymph in the labyrinth. Preventative management includes an avoid-salt diet and diuretics. Acute attacks are treated with meclizine 25 mg q6h po, diazepam 5 mg q4h po, or promethazine 12.5 to 25 mg q4h. For extreme symptoms, diazepam 5 mg i.v. will provide prompt improvement in severe dysphoria, nausea, vomiting, and immobilization.

Benign paroxysmal positional vertigo (BPPV) is caused by debris in the semicircular canals (mostly posterior canal) and leads to recurrent episodes lasting several hours to several days of intense positional vertigo. Patients do not experience deafness or tinnitus. Treatment should include an attempt to clear out the debris from the canal and into the vestibule (called the canalith repositioning maneuver or modified Epley maneuver). Repositioning is reported to work well in 70% to 80% of patients.

Acute labyrinthitis or vestibular neuronitis is a self-limited monophasic illness often seen in the setting of an upper respiratory infection. Vertigo from brainstem or cerebellar disease tends to be associated with other CNS symptoms/signs and related to TIA, stroke, multiple sclerosis (MS), or neoplasm. Additional conditions that should be considered in patients with chronic vertigo include syphilis, exposure to aminoglycoside antibiotics, and neurosarcoidosis.

Our patient's history of recurrent vertiginous dizziness and intermittent tinnitus would suggest an otologic or peripheral cause, most likely Ménière's disease. The rather persistent and frequent occurrence of symptoms is unusual for early Ménière's. Although classic Ménière's is associated with hearing loss and subjective fullness, some patients may not have the complete tetrad of symptoms. The presence of tinnitus and the absence of a striking positional trigger make benign positional vertigo less likely. The chronic nature of his symptoms is against viral vestibular neuronitis or labyrinthitis. His history of improvement associated with corticosteroid therapy raises the question of an inflammatory process such as a viral or immune-mediated etiology (such as neurosarcoidosis).

■ SELECTED REFERENCES

Baloh RW. Clinical practice. Vestibular neuritis. *N Engl J Med* 2003;348:1027–1032.
Biller J, ed. *Practical neurology,* 2nd ed. Philadelphia: Lippincott Williams & Wilkins, 2002.
Eggers SDZ, Zee DS. Evaluating the dizzy patient; bedside examination and laboratory assessment of the vestibular system. *Semin Neurol* 2003;23:47–58.
Epley JM. Human experience with canalith repositioning maneuvers. *Ann NY Acad Sci* 2001;942:179–191.

■ SEE QUESTIONS: 19, 64, 65

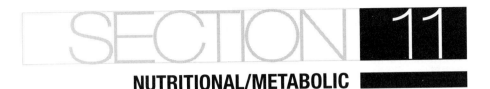

SECTION 11

NUTRITIONAL/METABOLIC

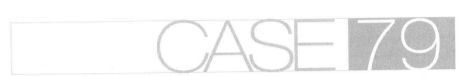

CASE 79

WERNICKE'S ENCEPHALOPATHY SECONDARY TO HYPEREMESIS GRAVIDARUM

OBJECTIVES

- To review the clinical manifestations and differential diagnosis of Wernicke's encephalopathy.
- To summarize the basic neuropathological findings of Wernicke's encephalopathy.
- To list the most frequent conditions associated with Wernicke's encephalopathy.
- To review management guidelines for Wernicke's encephalopathy.

VIGNETTE

This 34-year-old woman had hyperemesis gravidarum in January 1999. At that time, she began to have intermittent oscillopsia and dizziness. She had gallbladder surgery in February 1999 and had induction of a stillborn child at 17 weeks of pregnancy.

CASE SUMMARY

Our patient had intractable vomiting due to hyperemesis gravidarum causing Wernicke's encephalopathy. Wernicke's encephalopathy results from a deficiency in vitamin B_1 or thiamine. A global confusional state (greater than 60%), ataxia predominantly of gait (50%), and a variety of ocular abnormalities (40%) are the hallmark of this condition. Ocular findings most commonly encountered are horizontal nystagmus, bilateral CN VI palsies, and conjugate gaze palsies, reflecting lesions of the vestibular nuclei, abducens nucleus, and paramedian pontine reticular formation.

Vertical gaze palsy reflecting compromise of the pretectum and periaqueductal gray is less common. Retinal hemorrhages and papilledema are rare. Pupillary abnormalities are encountered in less than 20% of patients. Vestibular paresis is uniformly present in the acute stage. The ataxia is predominantly cerebellar as a result of involvement of the superior cerebellar vermis and vestibular nuclei. Rarely, patients develop stupor, coma, or hypothermia.

Numerous conditions have been associated with Wernicke's encephalopathy including chronic alcoholism, starvation, hyperemesis gravidarum, gastrointestinal tract malignancies, lymphoid-hemopoietic malignancies, anorexia nervosa, hunger strikers, acquired immunodeficiency syndrome, pyloric stenosis, gastric stapling for morbid obesity, inappropriate parenteral nutrition, prolonged intravenous feeding, digitalis intoxication, chronic hemodialysis or long-standing peritoneal dialysis, drug treatment for obesity, and thyrotoxicosis.

Pathologically, there is evidence of bilateral symmetrical periventricular (third ventricle, aqueduct of Sylvius, and fourth ventricle) lesions in the brainstem and medial thalamus. The anterior cerebellar vermis is frequently involved, and atrophy of the mammillary bodies is seen in the majority of chronic cases. Affected structures show endothelial proliferation and the presence of microscopic petechial hemorrhages.

Diagnosis of Wernicke's encephalopathy is facilitated by MRI, which is more sensitive than CT in detecting the acute periventricular and diencephalic lesions as demonstrated in our patient. Differential diagnosis of patients presenting with confusion, ataxia, and oculomotor disturbances must include conditions such as drug intoxication, particularly sedatives and anticonvulsants, posterior fossa strokes, subacute meningitides, subdural hematoma, and Leigh's encephalomyelopathy. Management of Wernicke's encephalopathy includes the administration of parenteral thiamine, bed rest, nutritional supplements, and the avoidance of glucose without thiamine. With thiamine administration, the abducens and conjugate palsies and the acute confusion are generally reversible; however, horizontal nystagmus and ataxia resolve completely in only approximately 40% of cases.

In summary, Wernicke's encephalopathy is a preventable disease. Untreated, it carries a mortality of 10% to 20%. The major long term complication is Korsakoff's syndrome. Failure to diagnose Wernicke's encephalopathy remains a serious concern. Numerous autopsy studies corroborate the rare occurrence of the full classical clinical triad.

■ SELECTED REFERENCES

Charness ME, Simon RP, Greenberg DA. Ethanol and the nervous system. *N Engl J Med* 1989;321:442–454.

Reuler JB, Girard DE, Cooney TG. Wernicke's encephalopathy. *N Engl J Med* 1985;312:1035–1038.

■ SEE QUESTIONS: 166, 171

CASE 80

CEREBROTENDINOUS XANTHOMATOSIS

OBJECTIVES

- To review the main clinical features of cerebrotendinous xanthomatosis (CTX) in a patient free of neurological manifestations.
- To review some diagnostic pitfalls in the diagnosis of CTX.
- To review ancillary diagnostic criteria for CTX.
- To discuss management strategies of CTX.

VIGNETTE

A 53-year-old hypertensive woman had a history of multiple "lumps" involving hands, knees, feet, and legs since age 9 and has had more than 400 operations to remove these lesions. She has experienced three heart attacks and had a CABG 7 years ago. She has not had any neurological complaints except for some blurry vision. She wears glasses. She has three living brothers, eight living sisters, and two daughters. There is a history of heart disease in one brother (deceased). Two brothers have had similar lumps.

On examination, her blood pressure was 138/72 mm Hg. She had bilateral carotid bruits and a grade II/VI systolic ejection murmur. In the conjunctiva, there was a large pterygium nasally extending very close to the visual axis of the right eye. She had a dense arcus of both corneas. In the fundus, the appearance of the disc, maculae, vessels, and periphery was normal. She had mild bilateral lens cataracts.

CASE SUMMARY

Our patient presented with pain around multiple xanthomatous lesions of the extremities. She stated that over 400 surgeries had been done since the age of 9. Initially she carried a diagnosis of neurofibromatosis and subsequently a diagnosis of phytosterolemia. Her examination showed numerous xanthomas present throughout her extremities. There were faint bilateral carotid bruits. Neurologic examination was normal. Carotid ultrasound showed 16% to 59% bilateral internal carotid artery stenosis.

MRI showed evidence of focal parietal atrophy but was otherwise unremarkable. MRS showed a mild increase in the N-acetylaspartate peak along with mild increased choline and lipid peaks. Serum cholesterol was 186 and serum cholestanol was elevated at 1.57 mg/dL (normal 0.2 ± 0.2 mg/dL). Urine was positive for tetrahydroxy, pentahydroxy, and hexahydroxy bile acid glucuronides, which is specific for sterol 27-hydroxylase deficiency. Cultured fibroblasts were checked for 27-sterol hydroxylase deficiency. The patient was switched from cholestyramine to colesevelam and started on azylamide and chenodeoxycholic acid (CDCA).

Cerebrotendinous xanthomatosis (CTX, Van Bogaert's disease) is a rare autosomal recessive lipid storage disorder caused by a mutation of the gene encoding the mitochondrial enzyme sterol 27-hydroxylase. It typically presents as a slowly progressive ataxia in conjunction with tendinous xanthomas. Pyramidal and cerebellar manifestations along with dementia are the predominant neurological manifestations. The xanthomas may also be seen in the quadriceps, triceps, and fingers in addition to the Achilles tendons, or they may be absent. Thickening of the interatrial septum compatible with lipomatous hypertrophy has been described in a few patients with CTX. Elevated serum cholestanol and urine bile acid glucuronides help to confirm the diagnosis.

The primary treatment of CTX is chenodeoxycholic acid (CDCA). HMG-CoA reductase inhibitors have also been used.

■ SELECTED REFERENCES

Dotti MT, Mondillo S, Plewina K, et al. Cerebrotendinous xanthomatosis: evidence of lipomatous hypertrophy of the atrial septum. *J Neurol* 1998;245:723–726.

Kuriyama M, Tokimura Y, Fujiyama J, et al. Treatment of cerebrotendinous xanthomatosis: effects of chenodeoxycholic acid, pravastatin, and combined use. *J Neurol Sci* 1994;125(Aug):22–28.

Schimschook JR, Alvord ECJ, Swanson PD. Cerebrotendinous xanthomatosis: clinical and pathologic studies. *Arch Neurol* 1968;18:688–698.

Van Bogaert L, et al. *Une forme cérébrale de la cholestérinose généralise.* Paris: Mason et Cie, 1937.

■ SEE QUESTION: 251

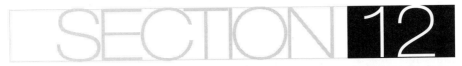

SECTION 12

HEADACHES/PAIN

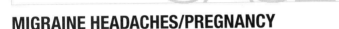

CASE 81

MIGRAINE HEADACHES/PREGNANCY

OBJECTIVES

- To review common and serious headache disorders occurring in pregnancy.
- To list the treatment options for migraine in pregnancy.

VIGNETTE

A 35-year-old woman, G2, P1, 36-week gestation, was evaluated because of recurrent headaches.

CASE SUMMARY

This patient presents with headache during pregnancy. Patients with episodic headache, throbbing or pounding quality, associated visual aura, intolerance of lights and noise, and nausea are typically diagnosed with migraine. The relationship between migraine and estrogen is well known including the tendency for migraine to occur around menses, to be aggravated by oral contraceptive medication, to develop following removal of the ovaries, and occurrence during pregnancy. Some women experience a reduction of migraine during and after menopause, whereas others begin to experience migraine in this setting. Similarly, pregnancy can be associated with a dramatic improvement in migraine for some women, especially those who have perimenstrual headaches, although others experience prominent migraine during pregnancy.

Commonly migraine begins occurring early in the second trimester. Management of migraine in pregnancy is problematic as many of the standard drugs used for prevention and those used for acute management are relatively contraindicated.

In general, acetaminophen is acceptable for PRN use in pregnancy. For more se-vere headaches acetaminophen with codeine is used. Beta-blockers (propranolol), verapamil, valproate, and tricyclic antidepressants are best avoided. Triptans and di-hydroergotamine should also be avoided except in extreme circumstances. At times headache severity and frequency are so severe as to require an open discussion with the patient, her neurologist, and her obstetrician and consider the risks and benefits of exposure to one of the drugs just named.

Serious causes of headache important to consider when evaluating a pregnant patient include intracranial venous or sinus thrombosis, pseudotumor cerebri, stroke, tumor, and severe preeclampsia, and if the headache develops abruptly, subarachnoid or intracerebral hemorrhage. Intracerebral hemorrhage is 2.5 times more likely during pregnancy and 28 times more likely during the first 6 weeks postpartum. The risk of aneurysmal subarachnoid hemorrhage is greatest during the third trimester, whereas arteriovenous malformations (AVMs) may be slightly more likely to bleed in the second trimester.

■ SELECTED REFERENCES

Biller J, ed. *Practical neurology* 2nd ed. Philadelphia: Lippincott Williams & Wilkins, 2002.
Roos KL, ed. *Headache and pregnancy.* In: *Neurologic disorders and pregnancy.* Continuum, Philadelphia 2000:114–127.

■ SEE QUESTIONS: 90, 134, 145, 146, 147, 260

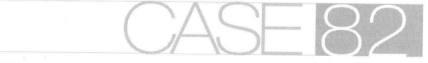

CLUSTER HEADACHES

OBJECTIVES

▦ To analyze the characteristic clinical features of episodic cluster headache.
▦ To briefly review the current classification of the many varieties of cluster headache.
▦ To summarize management guidelines for episodic cluster headache.

VIGNETTE

A 28-year-old man was evaluated because of recurrent unilateral headaches.

CASE SUMMARY

Without any warnings, our patient experienced a rather stereotypical syndrome characterized by recurrent brief attacks of severe unilateral pain centered around the left periorbital/retroorbital region, lasting 60 to 90 minutes. The pain was constant and more common at night, awakening him from sleep. He had no gastrointestinal complaints. During the attacks, he would become restless, unable to lie flat, having to constantly pace around.

There were ipsilateral autonomic signs related to sympathetic paresis and parasympathetic system overactivity such as conjunctival injection, lacrimation, rhinorrhea, and eyelid ptosis and miosis (as noted on his medical records). He had no manifestations of trigeminal nerve dysfunction. The attacks occurred with a frequency from once daily to once every other day, lasting for a few weeks to 2 months. There was a characteristic periodicity with pain-free intervals of many years. High-flow oxygen therapy was very effective in aborting an attack.

According to the International Headache Society (IHS), our patient fulfilled diagnostic criteria for episodic cluster headache. Cluster headache has been classified into (i) episodic, (ii) chronic, (iii) chronic paroxysmal hemicrania, and (iv) cluster headachelike syndrome. Chronic cluster headaches have been further subdivided into primary chronic (chronic from onset) and secondary chronic (chronic cluster headache evolving from episodic cluster headache). Eighty percent of cluster sufferers have the episodic variety of cluster. Men are affected more than women (6:1 ratio). The exact prevalence of cluster headache is unknown but has been estimated to be at least 0.4% in men and 0.08% in women.

Periodicity is a main feature of episodic cluster headache, with the cluster period lasting 2 to 3 months, and has been attributed to hypothalamic influences. Typical attacks often occur at the same time each day, awakening patients from sleep. They usually last between 15 to 30 minutes up to 180 minutes and occur with a frequency from once every other day to eight a day. Cluster periods typically occur every 1 to 2 years. Chronic cluster headaches refers to typical cluster headaches whose cycle is longer than 6 months without remission or with remissions lasting less than 2 weeks. In chronic paroxysmal hemicrania, the attacks are considerably shorter (5 to 45 minutes) than in episodic cluster headache and also more frequent (7 to 22 per day).

Chronic paroxysmal hemicrania is more common among women and is responsive to indomethacin. Symptomatic forms of cluster headache or cluster headachelike syndrome have been described in association with a variety of lesions, usually near the cavernous sinus, including tumors (e.g., parasellar meningiomas, pituitary adenomas, nasopharyngeal carcinomas), vascular malformations, carotid and vertebral artery aneurysms, and giant cell arteritis among others. Symptomatic clusterlike headaches should be suspected if there is a lack of periodicity to the patient's complaints, if there is residual background pain between pain clusters, if the neurologic examination is abnormal besides ptosis and miosis, or if traditional therapy is ineffective.

Management of episodic cluster headache may be symptomatic/abortive or prophylactic/preventive. Precise documentation of potential drug contraindications and potential drug interactions must be taken into consideration when selecting among the many available pharmacologic agents. The most effective symptomatic treatment of cluster headache is inhalation of high-flow concentrated oxygen, 6 to 8 L per min by face mask, for no longer than 20 minutes. Other abortive strategies include the intranasal administration of 4% lidocaine, subcutaneous sumatriptan, sublingual or inhaled ergotamine, and injectable dihydroergotamine (DHE 45 injection) preparations.

The prophylactic treatment of episodic cluster headaches includes verapamil, ergotamine, lithium carbonate, methysergide, prednisone, divalproex, and topiramate. Verapamil is the most effective calcium channel blocker for cluster headache prophylaxis and the treatment of first choice. Methysergide should not be given continuously for more than 6 months; a drug-free interval of 4 weeks must follow each course. Potentially devastating effects of methysergide include retroperitoneal, endocardial, and pulmonary fibrosis. Combined therapy is often necessary and may be very effective. Patients should avoid alcohol.

■ SELECTED REFERENCES

Biller J, ed. *Practical neurology,* 2nd ed. Philadelphia: Lippincott Williams & Wilkins, 2002.

Headache Classification Committee of the International Headache Society. Classification and diagnostic criteria for headache disorders, cranial neuralgias and facial pain. *Cephalagia* 1988;8[Suppl 7]:9–96.

Kudrow L. *Cluster headache: mechanisms and management.* London: Oxford University Press, 1980.

Kudrow L. The pathogenesis of cluster headache. *Curr Opin Neurol* 1994;7:278–282.

■ SEE QUESTIONS: 133, 134, 135, 136, 144, 145, 146, 147, 259

CASE 83

CSF HYPOTENSION SYNDROME

OBJECTIVES

■ To analyze the characteristic clinical and neuroimaging features of spontaneous intracranial hypotension syndrome.

■ To summarize management guidelines for spontaneous intracranial hypotension syndrome.

VIGNETTE

A 49-year-old previously healthy woman was admitted for evaluation of new-onset headaches.

CASE SUMMARY

Without an apparent precipitating factor such as head trauma, back trauma, or lumbar puncture, our patient experienced incapacitating positional headaches. Headaches were worse on assuming a sitting or standing position relative to supine or prone. Headaches were refractory to analgesics including codeine. She then developed horizontal diplopia. She had no fever, neck stiffness, CSF rhinorrhea, or upper extremity radicular complaints. Eventually, a brain MRI showed diffuse thickening of the pachymeninges with abnormal intense enhancement with gadolinium. She was initially erroneously suspected of having meningitis, and when a lumbar puncture (LP) was attempted, she was told she had a "dry tap." She was then referred for further evaluation.

On her initial examination, she was afebrile and only had mild limitation of abduction of the right eye. A radionuclide cisternogram showed asymmetric activity projecting in the right posterior lateral region of the cervical spine. A cervical CT myelogram showed abnormal epidural collections of contrast focally at C2-C3 anteriorly and C5-C6 posterolaterally. There was also bilateral C7-T1 and T1-T2 epidural contrast extending through the neural foramina and surrounding bilateral root sleeves and ganglia. These findings were more pronounced at C7-T1 on the left. After bed rest, administration of intravenous fluids, and two autologous epidural blood patches, she had marked recovery with complete resolution of her headaches and diplopia. Within 3 months, she became asymptomatic and returned to work full time.

Our patient had the cardinal features of spontaneously occurring intracranial hypotension. The most common symptom of spontaneous intracranial hypotension is an orthostatic holocranial headache, similar to headaches after lumbar puncture. Relief of pain by lying flat is characteristic. Straining and coughing exacerbate the pain. The onset of headaches may be sudden or gradual. Patients may also complain of neck or interscapular pain, nausea, vomiting, diplopia, visual blurring, facial numbness, dysgeusia, decreased hearing, tinnitus, dizziness, faintness when standing, and upper limb radicular symptoms. Minimal neck stiffness may be present. Typical MRI features consist of diffuse pachymeningeal enhancement following the administration of gadolinium, thought to represent engorgement of the dural vasculature.

The ventricles may be slitlike. There may be evidence of brain descent, including descent of the cerebellar tonsils and tight basilar cisterns. Subdural collections (hematomas and hygromas) have been described. Enlargement of the pituitary gland has been described. By definition, the CSF pressure is low (60 mm H_2O or less) or unobtainable, and there is no history of previous dural puncture. However, some patients with spontaneous intracranial hypotension have normal CSF pressure; this suggests that CSF hypovolemia rather than hypotension may play a pathogenic role. The CSF composition is usually normal, but there may be slight CSF protein elevation, a variable lymphocytic pleocytosis, and few red blood cells. A thorough investigation to test for CSF leaks along the neuraxis should be undertaken.

A CSF leak is documented in most, if not all, cases of spontaneous intracranial hypotension, usually at the level of the cervicothoracic junction or thoracic spine. MRI of the spine may demonstrate the level of the CSF leak or associated meningeal diverticula or dilated epidural veins in the high cervical region. CT myelogram of the entire spine may be necessary. Management involves bed rest, oral or intravenous fluids, oral or intravenous caffeine therapy, analgesics, steroids, and the administration of autologous epidural blood patches or continuous epidural saline infusions. Many patients require repair of the CSF leak. The MRI findings of meningeal enhancement diminish or disappear as clinical symptoms subside. The prognosis is generally favorable. Most patients can be cured after a correct diagnosis is made.

■ SELECTED REFERENCES

Bell WE, Joynt RJ, Sahs AL. Low spinal fluid pressure syndromes. *Neurology* 1961;10:512–521.

Mokri B, Piepgras DG, Miller GM. Syndrome of orthostatic headaches and diffuse pachymeningeal gadolinium enhancement. *Mayo Clin Proc* 1997;72:400–413.

Mokri B, Posner JB. Spontaneous intracranial hypotension. The broadening clinical and imaging spectrum of CSF leaks. Neurology 2000;55:1771–1772.

Pannullo SC, Reich JB, Krol G, et al. MRI changes in intracranial hypotension. *Neurology* 1993;43:919–926.

■ SEE QUESTIONS: 96, 97, 136, 137, 144, 145, 151, 154, 162, 258

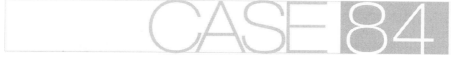

PSEUDOTUMOR CEREBRI

OBJECTIVES

- To describe criteria for the diagnosis of pseudotumor cerebri.
- To describe potential causes of pseudotumor cerebri.
- To discuss the differential diagnosis of bilateral optic disc edema.
- To review treatment guidelines for patients with pseudotumor cerebri.

VIGNETTE

A 31-year-old woman was evaluated because of headaches.

CASE SUMMARY

This young obese normotensive woman presented with a combination of long-standing headaches, visual scotomata, bilateral papilledema, and enlarged blind spots on visual field testing. She was not receiving oral contraceptives. Visual acuity was 20/20

OU. The remainder of her neurological examination was unremarkable. Neuroimaging investigations showed a normal brain MRI and normal magnetic resonance venography (MRV). Having excluded an intracranial mass or cerebral venous thrombosis as the etiology of the papilledema, she had a lumbar puncture, which showed elevated opening pressure and normal CSF composition.

A diagnosis of pseudotumor cerebri was made. As there was no known exposure to exogenous substances associated with pseudotumor cerebri and her visual acuity was preserved, her initial management consisted of a weight reduction diet, symptomatic headache treatment, and acetazolamide 500 mg twice daily.

The diagnosis of pseudotumor cerebri, also known as idiopathic intracranial hypertension, or benign intracranial hypertension, includes the following criteria: (i) symptoms and signs of raised intracranial pressure (headaches, transient visual obscurations, and horizontal diplopia due to unilateral or bilateral CN VI palsy), (ii) normal neuroimaging studies (MRI and MRV preferably; MRI may show small ventricles and occasionally an empty sella), and (iii) increased opening CSF pressure (greater than 250 mm H_2O) with normal composition (may show a low CSF protein). Patients may also complain of pulsatile tinnitus. Occasionally patients may present with oculomotor or trochlear nerve palsies or skew deviation.

Most common in obese young women, pseudotumor cerebri has been associated with a variety of exogenous substances including tetracyclines, nalidixic acid, amiodarone, corticosteroids, danazol, lithium, hypervitaminosis A, cyclosporine, indomethacin, growth hormone, and so on. Infants seem more susceptible to tetracyclines. Pseudotumor cerebri has also been reported in association with corticosteroid withdrawal, pregnancy, menarche, systemic lupus erythematosus (SLE) and other systemic diseases, hypoparathyroidism, thyroid replacement, high-flow arteriovenous malformations, radical neck dissection and other disorders of cerebral venous drainage. Although less frequent, pseudotumor cerebri occur in men as well.

Differential diagnosis of patients presenting with bilateral swollen optic discs should always encompass papilledema due an intracranial mass lesion, papillitis, anterior ischemic optic neuropathy (AION), pseudopapilledema, optic nerve head drusen, bilateral optic nerve tumors, and malignant hypertension. MRI and MRV should be obtained to rule out an intracranial mass lesion or cerebral venous thrombosis. CSF studies are needed to exclude inflammatory/infectious disorders or leptomeningeal malignancy.

Uncontrolled papilledema may result in progressive peripheral visual field constriction or nerve fiber bundle defects. The goal of treatment is visual preservation and consists of weight loss for those patients who are overweight and diuretics such as acetazolamide or furosemide. For those patients who have deterioration of their visual function related to optic nerve dysfunction, surgical treatment consists of optic nerve sheath fenestration or lumboperitoneal shunt.

■ SELECTED REFERENCES

Brazis PW, Lee AG. Elevated intracranial presure and pseudotumor cerebri. *Curr Opin Ophthalmol* 1998;9(6):27–32.

Corbett JJ, Savino PJ, Thompson HS, et al. Visual loss in pseudotumor cerebri. Follow-up of 57 patients from five to 41 years and a profile of 14 patients with permanent severe visual loss. *Arch Neurol* 1982;39:461–474.

Digre KB, Corbett JJ. *Practical viewing of the optic disc.* Boston: Butterworth-Heineman, 2003.

■ SEE QUESTIONS: 145, 146, 160, 161, 162

CASE 85

TRIGEMINAL NEURALGIA

OBJECTIVES

■ To present a typical patient with idiopathic trigeminal neuralgia (tic douloureux).
■ To review relevant applied anatomy of the trigeminal nerve (CN V).
■ To review management guidelines for patients with trigeminal neuralgia.

VIGNETTE

A 48-year-old man complained of episodic bursts of sharp, shooting left-sided facial pain.

CASE SUMMARY

This middle-aged man presented with multiple episodes of severe, brief (few seconds), stabbing, unilateral (left-sided only) facial pain, affecting predominantly the dermatomal zones innervated by the maxillary (V2) and mandibular (V3) branches of the trigeminal nerve (CN V), and to a lesser extent the dermatomal zone innervated by the ophthalmic (V1) branch. The episodes of pain were frequently triggered by painless sensory stimuli such as a draft of cold wind, chewing, or even a kiss. The episodes were repetitive, usually three to four in a given day. Between attacks, he had no symptoms. Neurological examination was normal.

Our patient provided an accurate description of a paroxysmal unilateral painful condition, with periods of remission, affecting the trigeminal nerve and typical of trigeminal neuralgia. The nucleus of the trigeminal nerve stretches from the midbrain (mesencephalic nucleus) through the pons (principal sensory and motor nucleus of V) to the upper cervical spinal cord region (nucleus of the spinal tract of the trigeminal nerve), where it becomes continuous with Lissauer's tract. The nucleus of the spinal tract of the trigeminal nerve is divided into a pars oralis, a pars interpolaris, and a pars caudalis.

The trigeminal nerve (CN V), the largest of the cranial nerves, exits laterally at the level of the midpons and its three divisions—ophthalmic (V1), maxillary (V2), and mandibular (V3)—proceed toward the gasserian ganglion located in Meckel's cave. From there the ophthalmic division (V1) exits the cranium via the superior orbital fissure, the maxillary division (V2) exits through the foramen rotundum, and the mandibular division (V3) exits via the foramen ovale. The trigeminal nerve provides sensory innervation of the face and supplies the muscles of mastication.

Trigeminal neuralgia (tic douloureux or Fothergill's disease) is the most frequent type of facial neuralgia. More common with advanced age, trigeminal neuralgia affects women more commonly than men. The most commonly affected dermatomal zones are innervated by V2 and V3 together. This pattern is more common than involvement of V2 or V3 alone. The V1 dermatome is the least affected. The right side tends to be affected more commonly than the left. The appearance of trigeminal neuralgia in a young patient should raise the suspicion of multiple sclerosis, in which it is often bilateral.

The pathogenesis of idiopathic trigeminal neuralgia is uncertain. Many cases of idiopathic trigeminal neuralgia may be due to pulsations of an aberrant vascular loop causing an area of demyelination of the trigeminal nerve root. Secondary forms of trigeminal neuralgia may be due to mass lesions or inflammation. Pontine demyelinating lesions at the root entry zone of the trigeminal nerve have been demonstrated in multiple sclerosis patients with trigeminal neuralgia.

The diagnosis of trigeminal neuralgia is purely clinical; diagnosis is usually made by history alone. As in our patient, the neurological examination findings are normal in idiopathic trigeminal neuralgia. An MRI is obtained to exclude an intracranial lesion that can result in pain resembling trigeminal neuralgia.

Medical management of patients with trigeminal neuralgia should be attempted first. Carbamazepine is the most effective medication. Other alternatives include oxcarbazepine, phenytoin, valproic acid, baclofen, gabapentin, lamotrigine, or clonazepam. If medical therapy is not successful, surgical therapy should be entertained. One of the most effective procedures is the microvascular decompression (Janetta procedure) of vascular elements from the trigeminal nerve. Percutaneous procedures include radiofrequency rhizotomy, glycerol rhizotomy, and balloon microcompression. An increasingly popular noninvasive outpatient procedure is stereotactic gamma knife radiosurgery.

■ SELECTED REFERENCES

Barker FG, Janetta PJ, Bissonette DJ. The long-term outcome of microvascular decompression for trigeminal neuralgia. *N Engl J Med* 1996;334:1077–1083.

Biller J, ed. *Practical neurology,* 2nd ed. Philadelphia: Lippincott Williams & Wilkins, 2002.

Burchile KV, Slavin KV. On the natural history of trigeminal neuralgia. *Neurosurgery* 2000;46:152–154.

Tenser RB. Trigeminal neuralgia: mechanisms of treatment. *Neurology* 1998;51(Jul):17–19.

■ SEE QUESTIONS: 62, 63, 133, 134, 146, 177

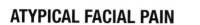

ATYPICAL FACIAL PAIN

OBJECTIVES

- To analyze the clinical features of atypical facial pain.
- To review the differential diagnosis of atypical facial pain.
- To summarize management guidelines for patients with atypical facial pain.

VIGNETTE

A 47-year-old woman complained of refractory constant left-sided facial pain of 8 years duration. Neurological examination was normal.

CASE SUMMARY

Our patient was a middle-aged woman who had an 8-year history of a predominantly unilateral and continuous left-sided facial pain that did not follow the anatomical boundaries of the trigeminal nerve. The pain was characterized as a deep aching and burning on the left side of her face, ear, and lateral aspect of her neck. Occasionally, it was described as sharp and or shooting. The pain was not aggravated by chewing, talking, touching the face at a specific point (trigger point), or lateral movements of the jaw. There was no history of odontalgia. She had no ipsilateral conjunctival injection or nasal congestion. She did not have nausea, photophobia, or sonophobia. Due to the almost continuous nature of her deep and intense facial pain, she became very irritable and experienced numerous mood swings. However, sleep was not affected.

She saw a variety of medical specialists. Initially she was thought to have a sinus infection. Then she was diagnosed with trigeminal neuralgia. Treatment with carbamazepine was unsuccessful. The diagnosis of trigeminal neuralgia was subsequently rejected by a neurosurgeon whom she consulted for a peripheral block by means of alcohol injections. Eventually, she had all her teeth removed without any benefit. Besides carbamazepine, numerous medications including tricyclic antidepressants, nonopioid analgesics, and finally opioid analgesics were tried but without satisfactory results. Neurologic and physical examination were normal. She had no trigger points. The temporomandibular joints were normal. There was no tenderness on palpation of the supraorbital and infraorbital foramina.

Based on her history of unrelenting facial pain with ill-defined anatomical boundaries, and after extensive investigations that excluded other possible structural causes of protracted facial pain, our patient was diagnosed with atypical facial pain. Despite its wide clinical acceptance as a separate entity, there are no well-accepted diagnostic criteria of atypical facial pain. The general characteristics of atypical facial pain

resemble those described by our patient. Although mostly unilateral, a bilateral occurrence is not rare. The cause of atypical facial pain remains unknown. Atypical
facial pain must be distinguished from trigeminal neuralgia (tic douloureux), temporomandibular joint syndrome, migraines, cluster headaches, temporal arteritis,
postherpetic neuralgia, odontalgia, neoplastic processes of the maxillary sinus or na-
sopharynx, and pain of psychological origin.

Management of patients with atypical facial pain is challenging. Pharmacologic
interventions include tricyclic antidepressants, gabapentin, lamotrigine, clonazepam,
transcutaneous nerve stimulation, sphenopalatine ganglion block, psychotherapy, and
behavioral approaches. After many strategies of pharmacologic combinations were
attempted without major success, a combination of gabapentin and the synthetic
prostaglandin E1 analog misoprostol (Cytotec) has decreased our patient's pain to
tolerable levels, improving her quality of life.

■ SELECTED REFERENCES

Biller J, ed. *Practical neurology,* 2nd ed. Philadelphia: Lippincott Williams & Wilkins, 2002.
Reder AT, Arnason BG. Trigeminal neuralgia in multiple sclerosis relieved by a prostaglandin E analogue. *Neurology* 1995;45:1097–1100.
Reik L. Atypical facial pain: a reappraisal. *Headache* 1985;25:30–32.
Turp J, Gobetti JP. Trigeminal neuralgia versus atypical facial pain: a review of the literature and case report. *Oral Surg, Oral Med, Oral Path, Oral Radiol Endod* 1996;81:424–432.

■ SEE QUESTIONS: 63, 133, 134, 159, 177

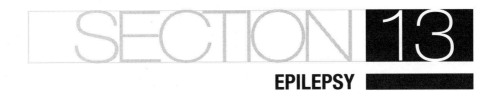

CASE 87

PARTIAL COMPLEX SEIZURES

OBJECTIVES

- To review the general classification of epilepsy.
- To describe the localizing signs of partial seizures.
- To describe the common treatment options of complex partial seizures.

VIGNETTE

An 18-year-old man was evaluated because of recurrent "spells" since the age of 11.

CASE SUMMARY

Our patient was an 18-year-old man with a history of complex partial and secondarily generalized seizures. He has had seizures since age 11. His seizures have been refractory to topiramate, oxcarbazepine, and levetiracetam. While being monitored in a video EEG room, this patient had a complex partial seizure. During the ictal phase, he had the sudden onset of a motionless stare and became unresponsive. Next, an abducting posture of both hands was noted and initially his right hand was held in a dystonic posture. Some mild lip smacking was noted. He then became restless with some purposeless hand movements. No sustained gaze deviation was noted. During the postictal phase, he probably had difficulty speaking, suggesting postictal dysphasia. A complex automatism was noted in his attempt to use the remote control.

An epileptic seizure is a transient and reversible alteration of behavior caused by a paroxysmal, abnormal, and excessive neuronal discharge. Epilepsy is typically defined as two or more recurring seizures not provoked by such triggers as intracranial infections, drug withdrawal, acute metabolic changes, or fever. Epileptic seizures are classified into two broad categories: partial (focal) seizures and generalized seizures. Partial seizures start in specific locations in the cerebral cortex and are often associated with focal ictal and interictal changes during an EEG. Generalized seizures are characterized by generalized involvement of the brain from the beginning of the seizure and have no consistent focal areas of ictal onset.

Partial seizures can become secondarily generalized tonic-clonic seizures. Partial seizures are further subdivided into simple partial and complex partial seizures. Consciousness remains intact during a simple partial seizure whereas consciousness is impaired during a complex partial seizure. Complex partial seizures are the most common seizure type in adults, and the temporal lobe, particularly the medial temporal lobe, is the most common site of the epileptogenic focus. There appears to be a strong relationship between complicated febrile seizures during early childhood or infancy and the later development of medial temporal lobe epilepsy. Lateralizing signs can often predict the side of abnormality or epileptogenic region in patients with partial epilepsy.

Forced and sustained head deviation and dystonic posturing of the upper extremity often indicate a contralateral epileptogenic region. Unilateral upper extremity automatisms may predict an ipsilateral seizure focus. Postictal dysphasia usually indicates a dominant-hemisphere seizure. This patient's ictal and postictal behavior would suggest a left temporal lobe focus.

The temporal lobe is the most common site of origin for partial seizures. Mesial temporal sclerosis is the most common abnormality seen on MRI images of the brain in patients with temporal lobe epilepsy. The patient's MRI shows evidence of left mesial temporal sclerosis and cortical dysplasia of the right anterior temporal region. His EEG showed frequent independent epileptiform discharges over both anterior midtemporal regions. His ictal single photon emission computed tomography (SPECT) scan during video EEG demonstrated hyperperfusion over the right temporal region. Subsequent positron emission tomography (PET) scan showed no focal deficits.

The first-line treatment of complex partial seizures is medical therapy with any number of antiepileptic medications. They may need to be used in combinations. For patients with medically refractory complex partial seizures, surgical treatment should be considered. If, after extensive evaluation, a single epileptogenic focus is found that does not involve eloquent cortex, resective surgery may be an option. Resection of the medial temporal lobe is the most common surgical procedure for treatment of medically refractory complex partial seizures. Due to discordance between electrographic and neuroimaging data, our patient did not have surgery.

■ **SELECTED REFERENCES**

Biller J, ed. *Practical neurology,* 2nd ed. Philadelphia: Lippincott Williams & Wilkins, 2002.

Chee MWL, Kotagal P, Van Ness PC, et al. Lateralizing signs in intractable partial epilepsy: blinded multiple-observer analysis. *Neurology* 1993;43:2519–2525.

French JA, Williamson PD, Thadnai VM, et al. Characteristics of medial temporal lobe epilepsy. I. results of history and physical examination. *Ann Neurol* 1993;34:774–780.

■ **SEE QUESTIONS: 6, 7, 8, 9, 21, 22, 23, 24, 25, 98, 99, 100, 101, 198, 222, 224, 236, 237**

CASE 88

PARTIAL SEIZURES WITH ELEMENTARY SYMPTOMATOLOGY

OBJECTIVES

▓ To define simple partial seizures.
▓ To discuss the use of folic acid in women taking antiepileptic medications.
▓ To discuss the management of epilepsy in pregnancy.

VIGNETTE

A 33-year-old woman had two episodes of right arm and forearm jerking movements lasting 2 to 5 minutes in June of 1996. On September 13, 1996, she had an 18-hour episode of continuous jerking involving the lower abdomen and her right arm. On September 7, 1998, she had a 10-minute episode of jerking movements involving the right foot followed by loss of consciousness and postictal confusion. On October 3, 1998, she had another 10-minute episode characterized by right foot jerking movements. Since this event, she has had some difficulty with dexterity of her right foot and has experienced episodes of tripping while going upstairs. She had no history of perinatal problems, meningitis, or encephalitis.

CASE SUMMARY

The patient had the onset of simple partial seizures manifested by elementary motor (clonic) symptomatology. This initially affected only her right arm, but with her second spell, both her right arm and lower abdomen were involved. She stopped antiepileptic drug (AED) use for an attempted pregnancy. Her next spell consisted of a partial seizure (right foot) followed by secondary generalization of her seizure. Antiepileptic medications were restarted. After her last spell, she reported residual decreased dexterity of right foot movements.

Her examination shows a decreased rate of foot tapping on the right associated with brisk reflexes in the right leg. Her MRI of the brain shows two areas of increased signal in the left hemisphere near the central sulcus. The exact nature of these lesions has not been defined and they have not progressed on subsequent imaging. She desires another pregnancy.

Partial seizures start in specific locations in the cerebral cortex and are often associated with focal ictal and interictal changes during an EEG. Partial seizures can become secondarily generalized tonic-clonic seizures. Partial seizures are further subdivided into simple partial and complex partial seizures. Consciousness remains intact during a simple partial seizure whereas consciousness is impaired during a complex partial seizure. The patient's treatment consisted of antiepileptic medication. Although the exact medication is not specified, any number of medications could be used to treat simple partial epilepsy. The complicating factor in her treatment is her desire to become pregnant while continuing to take antiepileptic medications.

For women who require antiepileptic drugs during their reproductive years, several guidelines should be kept in mind. Whichever AED is deemed appropriate for the type of seizures can be used. Monotherapy should be the aim of therapy. Several AEDs, especially the enzyme-inducing ones, decrease the effectiveness of hormonal contraception. This should be discussed with the woman to avoid any unwanted pregnancies. All women of childbearing age taking AEDs should be taking folic acid at 1 to 4 mg per day. Folic acid supplementation lessens the chance of birth defects, especially neural tube defects. If a woman taking an AED desires a pregnancy and wishes to discontinue the AED (and it is clinically appropriate), conversion to monotherapy to the lowest effective dose should be considered.

A change to an alternative AED should not be undertaken during pregnancy for the sole purpose of reducing teratogenic risk. For women who are pregnant and taking an AED, prenatal testing with AFP levels at 14 to 16 weeks and fetal ultrasound at 16 to 20 weeks should be offered. If appropriate, amniocentesis for amniotic α-fetoprotein (AFP) levels can be done. This may be especially useful in patients taking carbamazepine, divalproex sodium, or valproic acid given the increased risk of neural tube defects noted with these medications. Close monitoring of AED levels during pregnancy and at least through the eighth week postpartum is necessary.

Changes in drug levels may be noted and adjustments to drug doses may be appropriate as weight changes and drug pharmacokinetic alterations occur during pregnancy. Vitamin K 10 mg per day should be given during the last month of pregnancy if the patient is taking enzyme-inducing AEDs. This is to prevent a hemorrhagic disease of the newborn because these AEDs can decrease the vitamin K–dependent clotting factors. If no oral vitamin K is given during the pregnancy, parenteral vitamin K should be given to the mother as soon as possible after the onset of labor. All neonates should receive vitamin K after delivery. Breast-feeding is not contraindicated, but one must be wary of neonatal sedation if the mother is taking sedating AEDs.

This patient followed the previous recommendations with fetal ultrasounds during pregnancy and frequent monitoring of AED levels. She also appropriately took Vitamin K. She had an uneventful pregnancy and delivered a healthy child.

■ SELECTED REFERENCES

Biller J, ed. *Practical neurology,* 2nd ed. Philadelphia: Lippincott Williams & Wilkins, 2002.
Practice parameter: management issues for women with epilepsy (summary statement from the Quality Standards Subcommittee of the American Academy of Neurology). Neurology 1998;51:944–948.

■ SEE QUESTIONS: 6, 7, 8, 9, 20, 21, 22, 23, 24, 25, 98, 99, 100, 101, 105, 198, 222, 226, 227, 236, 237, 238

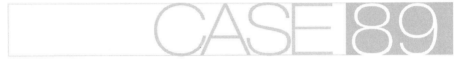

TUBEROUS SCLEROSIS COMPLEX

OBJECTIVES

- To review the main clinical manifestations of tuberous sclerosis complex (TSC).
- To discuss the genetic basis of TSC.
- To discuss the ancillary evaluation of patients with TSC.
- To summarize treatment guidelines for patients with TSC.

VIGNETTE

A 40-year-old man has had epileptic seizures since the age of 3 years.

CASE SUMMARY

Our patient had a history of mental retardation, epileptic seizures, and facial angiofibromas in a butterfly distribution over the nose, cheeks, and chin, characteristic of the tuberous sclerosis complex (TSC). TSC is inherited as an autosomal dominant trait, although the rate of spontaneous mutation is high. TSC has been identified in all races and in all parts of the world. Recently, two genes, TSC1 on chromosome 9, which encodes for the protein hamartin, and TSC2 on chromosome 16, which encodes for the protein tuberin, have been identified. TSC affects almost every organ system, most commonly the brain, skin, eyes, kidneys, heart, and lungs. The most common neurological manifestations are partial or generalized seizures including infantile spasms during the first years of life. Other neurological manifestations include mental retardation, hydrocephalus, autism, and pervasive developmental and other behavioral disorders.

The most commonly found CNS lesions are cortical tubers, subependymal nodules, and subependymal giant cell astrocytomas adjacent to the foramen of Monro. Common skin manifestations include ash-leaf spots or hypopigmented lesions (seen better with a Wood lamp), facial angiofibromas, shagreen patches (leathery plaque), and ungal and periungal fibromas (Koenen's tumors). Ocular manifestations include retinal hamartomas or astrocytomas and colobomas of the iris, lens, and choroid. Renal manifestations consist of angiomyolipomas and renal cysts; hematuria, arterial hypertension, and renal failure may develop in severe cases. Cardiac rhabdomyomas may be asymptomatic or cause outflow obstruction, abnormal valve function, or cardiac arrhythmias. The two most common lung lesions are pulmonary cysts and lymphangioleiomyomatosis; spontaneous pneumothorax is a rare complication.

An MRI of the brain is recommended for the evaluation and follow-up of cortical tubers, subependymal nodules, and subependymal giant cell astrocytomas. EEG may demonstrate hypsarrhythmia in an infant with infantile spasms. Funduscopic examination may show retinal hamartomas or astrocytomas. Echocardiography is indicated for the detection of cardiac rhabdomyomas. Renal changes can be demonstrated by renal ultrasound, CT, or MRI. Chest roentgenography or chest CT is indicated for the evaluation of lung lesions. Testing to determine genetic mutations with DNA probes is available at research centers. Epileptic seizures are treated with standard antiepileptic drugs. A ketogenic diet may be considered. Neurosurgery consultation may be required in cases of raised intracranial pressure.

■ SELECTED REFERENCES

Biller J, ed. *Practical neurology,* 2nd ed. Philadelphia: Lippincott Williams & Wilkins, 2002.

Roach ES, Gomez MR, Northrup H. Tuberous sclerosis complex consensus conference: revised clinical diagnostic criteria. *J Child Neurol* 1998;13:624–628.

Roach ES, Williams DP, Laster DW. Magnetic resonance imaging in tuberous sclerosis. *Arch Neurol* 1987;44:301–303.

■ SEE QUESTIONS: 6, 7, 8, 9, 21, 22, 23, 24, 25, 98, 99, 100, 101, 105, 142, 176, 198, 222, 224

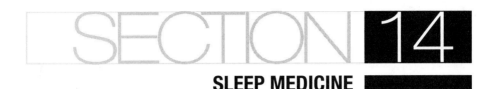

SECTION 14

SLEEP MEDICINE

CASE 90

OBSTRUCTIVE SLEEP APNEA

OBJECTIVES

▨ To review the common causes of excessive daytime sleepiness.
▨ To outline the treatment strategies for obstructive sleep apnea.
▨ To recognize the common features of narcolepsy.

VIGNETTE

A 71-year-old man with history of chronic obstructive pulmonary disease (COPD), atrial fibrillation, carotid stenosis, TIAs, secondary polycythemia, and essential tremor was evaluated because of excessive snoring. (The interview was conducted after the patient had received treatment for the underlying condition.)

CASE SUMMARY

The patient presents with excessive daytime sleepiness. Other than hypothyroidism, overmedication, metabolic encephalopathy, and depression the patient should be evaluated for a sleep disorder.

Sleep disorders are prevalent and underrecognized, they have costly implications, and they can be very serious, but fortunately, they are very treatable. For example, obstructive sleep apnea is estimated to be more prevalent than asthma. In 1990 in the United States there were 200,000 motor vehicle accidents as a result of falling sleep at the wheel. Nearly one-third of all heavy trucking accidents in which the driver is injured are due to the driver falling asleep at the wheel. A number of major industrial catastrophes, including the Exxon *Valdez*, Three Mile Island, and Chernobyl have been associated with sleepiness-related errors in judgment or performance in the workplace.

Thirty million Americans are estimated to suffer from chronic sleep disorders, of which 95% are considered to be underdiagnosed and untreated. In addition, another 20 or 30 million Americans are estimated to experience sleep-associated problems. A survey in 1990 suggested the direct cost of sleepiness and sleep disorders to the American public was $16 billion with indirect costs of $160 billion.

Obstructive sleep apnea (OSA) is a common syndrome classically presenting as excessive daytime sleepiness and fatigue. Additionally, patients are at risk for cardiovascular manifestations of chronic intermittent hypoxia (hypertension, pulmonary hypertension, arrhythmia, cor pulmonale). Patients are classically obese, often with underlying chronic pulmonary disease. Another group has anatomic problems with the upper airway leading to obstruction (large adenoids; palate and pharyngeal problems; short, stocky, muscular necks; small chins). Patients with OSA snore heavily. They are usually unaware of problems with nighttime sleep, but in fact have poor quality of sleep.

Presumably, the obstruction produces hypoxia, which interferes with achieving deep stages of sleep (hypoxia causes arousal). Patients wake up frequently for brief periods and never achieve adequate quantities of deep (stage III or IV) sleep. Occasionally they present with early-morning headaches due to hypercapnia and occasionally memory impairment or personality change due to hypoxia. Simple observation of sleep will make the diagnosis, but a nighttime sleep study will quantify the severity of obstruction and hypoxia. Therapy depends on the severity. Weight loss is an effective and simple therapeutic measure. Following diagnosis, most patients are treated with positive airway pressure to eliminate obstruction (biPAP).

Central sleep apnea is a less common and less well understood disorder with multiple causes usually related to disease of the brainstem respiratory centers. A polysomnogram is required to make this diagnosis and referral to neurology is necessary. Ondine's curse is perhaps the most severe form.

Narcolepsy is a tetrad of symptoms as follows:

1. Sleep attacks—more like irresistible naps that patients struggle to fight off.
2. Cataplexy—sudden loss of muscle tone without loss of consciousness provoked by a strong emotional stimulus. Laughing is the strongest emotional trigger of cataplexy.
3. Hypnagogic hallucinations—stereotyped vivid dreams while falling asleep or awakening (hypnopompic).
4. Sleep paralysis—common in the general population. Episodes of inability to move while falling asleep or waking, often frightening to the patient.

Narcolepsy has a hereditary basis. About 90% of narcoleptic patients have HLA DR2/DQ1 that is present in less than 30% of the general population. Recent studies indicate that hypocretin is markedly reduced in narcoleptics. The onset is variable, often in adolescence, and the evaluation requires a multiple sleep latency test (MSLT). This study is done in the EEG or sleep lab and consists of monitoring EEG and eye movements as the patient lies down in a dark room for five trials or naps in one day. The length of time required for the onset of EEG-confirmed sleep is averaged (the average sleep latency). This will document and quantify the degree of excessive daytime sleepiness. Most narcoleptics enter REM sleep within minutes of falling asleep. This finding usually establishes the diagnosis. These patients are managed with scheduled naps and usually prescribed CNS stimulants such as caffeine, amphetamine, and modafinil.

■ SELECTED REFERENCES

Barthlen GM. Sleep-disordered breathing. In: *Sleep Disorders:* Continuum, Philadelphia 2002;8:147–155.
Krahn LE, Black JL, Silber MH. Narcolepsy: new understanding of irresistible sleep. *Mayo Clinic Proc* 2001;76:185–194.

■ SEE QUESTIONS: 124, 125, 126, 130, 131, 132, 206

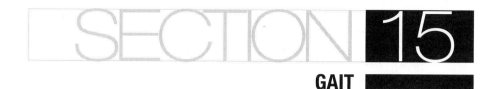

SECTION **15**

GAIT

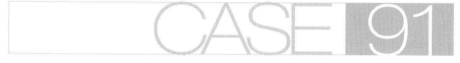

CASE 91

GAIT APRAXIA (MAGNETIC GAIT)

OBJECTIVES

▤ To present a patient with a diagnostically challenging gait disorder.
▤ To briefly review the clinical entity of normal pressure hydrocephalus (NPH).

VIGNETTE

A 76-year-old woman with a prior small vessel subcortical infarct was evaluated because of an inability to walk.

CASE SUMMARY

Our patient had a prior small subcortical infarct and consulted us because of her severe gait disability and frequent falling. She did not complain of headaches, nausea, vomiting, or visual difficulties. She had no history of subarachnoid hemorrhage, meningitis, cranial radiation, cranial surgery, or head trauma. Despite her severe gait disorder, our patient could move her legs fairly well, particularly when lying on her back. She did not have ataxia or overt muscle weakness.

Although she was able to stand, she had marked difficulty in lifting her feet and walked as if her feet were glued to the floor. Arm swing during walking was relatively preserved, and she did not have resting tremor, bradykinesia, or rigidity. Turning was difficult and it took several steps. Her gait difficulties and falling episodes continued despite a trial of levodopa/carbidopa. MRI did not show ventricular enlargement or leukoaraiosis. On T2 weighted images, there was no evidence of increased signal in the periventricular areas. There was no thinning or bowing of the corpus callosum. There was no prominent flow void noticed in the aqueduct and third ventricle. Isotope cisternography was reported as showing a mixed pattern.

Our patient has the so-called magnetic type of gait disorder. This type of gait disorder may be caused by bilateral lesions of the medial frontal cortex, bilateral ischemic lesions of the white matter, or severe hydrocephalus. Hydrocephalus may be due to disorders of CSF production, CSF circulation, or CSF absorption. Some forms of hydrocephalus cannot be properly classified according to that scheme, as is the case of normal pressure hydrocephalus (NPH). NPH is a clinical entity seen in older subjects and characterized by ventriculomegaly and normal CSF pressure.

NPH may occur after subarachnoid hemorrhage, meningitis, intracranial surgery, or head trauma, but in a large number of patients, the cause is unknown. NPH is characterized by progressive gait disturbance, dementia, and urinary incontinence. Gait impairment is the most prominent and often the earliest manifestation of NPH. Distinguishing the gait disorder encountered among patients with NPH from other disorders of gait encountered in older adults may be difficult.

The next diagnostic steps in our patient should include a baseline neuropsychological evaluation and a timed walking test. The patient should then have a large-volume lumbar puncture with measurement of the opening pressure and removal of approximately 50 cc of CSF, and the previous examinations should be repeated approximately 3 hours later. A clinical improvement of gait predicts a good response to shunting. However, selection of patients (suspected of having NPH) for shunting remains controversial. Infection, subdural hematomas, and shunt failure are feared complications of shunting.

■ SELECTED REFERENCES

Adams RD, Fisher CM, Hakim S, et al. Symptomatic occult hydrocephalus with "normal" cerebrospinal fluid pressure. A treatable syndrome. *N Engl J Med* 1965;273:117–126.

Vanneste J, Augustijn P, Dirven C, et al. Shunting normal pressure hydrocephalus: do the benefits outweigh the risks? *Neurology* 1992;42:54–59.

Wikkelso C, Anderson H, Blomstrand C, et al. Normal pressure hydrocephalus: predictive value of the cerebrospinal fluid tap-test. *Acta Neurol Scand* 1986;73:566–573.

■ SEE QUESTIONS: 160, 161

CASE 92

HEMIPLEGIC GAIT/SPASTICITY

OBJECTIVES

▥ To illustrate the disabilities associated with spasticity.
▥ To analyze the characteristic features of a spastic gait.
▥ To briefly summarize available management strategies for spasticity.

VIGNETTE

At the age of 39, this 46-year-old man with a history of hypertension, diabetes, hyperlipidemia, and obesity had a right subcortical infarct involving the posterior limb of the internal capsule. Further evaluation also demonstrated the presence of a paten foramen ovale and an atrial septal aneurysm.

CASE SUMMARY

Due to a right posterior limb of the internal capsule infarct with subsequent disruption of the corticospinal tract, our patient was left with a disabling spastic left hemiparesis. As a result of his spasticity, he had numerous complaints including inadequate use of his affected hand and leg, troubles walking, curling of his left toes, scraping of the floor with the outer edge of his left foot, callous formation of his left foot, pain, and occasional flexor spasms. In addition to his left hemiparesis involving his face, arm, and leg, he also had signs of spasticity characterized by increased muscle tone, clasp-knife phenomenon, hyperreflexia, clonus, and a Babinski sign (not shown on the tape). He had a characteristic spastic hemiparetic gait. There was spastic adduction and internal rotation of the left shoulder and a clenched left fist. The left leg was externally rotated at the hip. The left knee was extended and stiff, and the left foot was plantar flexed and inverted (equinovarus). He had a tendency to circumduct and scuffed the left foot.

Damage to the upper motor neurons results in muscles that are initially weak and flaccid, but eventually become spastic and exhibit hypertonia and hyperactivity of the stretch reflexes. *Spasticity* is defined as an increase in muscle tone due to hyperexcitability of the stretch reflex and is characterized by a velocity-dependent increase in tonic stretch reflexes. Spasticity can be cerebral or spinal in origin. Common causes of cerebral spasticity include cerebro-vascular disease, demyelinating disease, and cerebral palsy. Common causes of spasticity of spinal cord origin include cervical spondylotic myelopathy, traumatic spinal cord injury, demyelinating disease, tumoral myelopathies, spinal cord vascular malformations, nutritional myelopathies (cobalamin deficiency), and tropical spastic paraparesis (HTLV-1).

Spasticity predominates on the antigravity muscles (flexors of the upper extremities and extensors of the lower extremities). Weakness of the muscles of the upper extremity is most marked in deltoid, triceps, wrist extension, and finger extension. This predilection for involvement of the extensors and supinators explains the pronation and flexion tendencies of the upper extremity. The spastic wrist is flexed, and often it may have a radial deviation. Weakness of the muscles of the lower extremities is most marked in hip flexion, knee flexion, foot dorsiflexion, and eversion. Equinovarus is the most common pathologic posture of the foot.

Spasticity may be present even in cases of only minimal weakness. Certain pathologic reflexes and signs appear. One of the most common is the extensor plantar reflex or Babinski sign characterized by extension of the great toe and fanning of the other toes. Clonus can often be elicited at the ankle or wrist. The superficial reflexes (abdominal reflexes, cremasteric reflex in men) are absent or suppressed on the affected side. If the lesion occurs above the level of the pyramidal decussation, these signs will be detected on the opposite side of the body; if it occurs below the pyramidal decussation, the signs will be detected on the same side. A commonly used scale to assess the degree of spasticity is the modified Ashworth Scale.

A variety of strategies are available for the management of spasticity. Physical therapy is of paramount importance in these patients. Medications that are useful for the management of spasticity are the GABA agonist baclofen, tizanidine, and diazepam. Selected patients can benefit from injections of botulinus toxin, which inhibits the release of acetylcholine at the neuromuscular junction, into specific muscles. In paraplegic patients with severe and disabling spasticity, intrathecal baclofen administration may be useful in ameliorating severe spasticity and urinary urgency. One of the most effective neurosurgical treatments for spasticity is selective dorsal rhizotomy.

■ SELECTED REFERENCES

Biller J, ed. *Practical neurology,* 2nd ed. Philadelphia: Lippincott Williams & Wilkins, 2002.

Brazis PW, Masdeu JC, Biller J. *Localization in clinical neurology,* 4th ed. Philadelphia: Lippincott Williams & Wilkins, 2001.

Lance JW. Symposium synopsis. In: Feldman RG, Yound RR, Koella WP, eds. *Spasticity: disordered motor control.* Chicago: 1980:485–494.

Simpson DM, Alexander DN, O'Brien CF, et al. Botulinum toxin A in the treatment of upper extremity spasticity: a randomized, double blind placebo controlled trial. *Neurology* 1996;46:1306–1310.

■ SEE QUESTIONS: 30, 55, 87

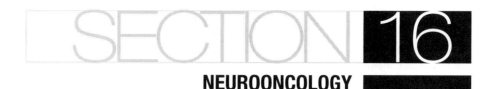

SECTION 16

NEUROONCOLOGY

CASE 93

LEPTOMENINGEAL MALIGNANCY (LYMPHOMA)

OBJECTIVES

- To recognize the presentation and manifestations of leptomeningeal malignancy.
- To outline the appropriate differential diagnosis and diagnostic workup for a chronic progressive polyradiculopathy and mononeuritis multiplex.
- To illustrate classic cerebrospinal fluid findings in leptomeningeal malignancy.
- To emphasize the importance of a thorough diagnostic workup for patients with progressive polyradiculopathy and mononeuritis multiplex.

VIGNETTE

A 38-year-old man presented with a subacute progressive afebrile illness characterized by right thigh numbness and itching followed by right lower back pain, left foot numbness and itching, left lower extremity burning pains, left hand numbness, and deep left elbow and upper back pain. Subsequently, he had tingling of his right toes and left-hand severe stabbing pains. More recently, he had left arm and right thigh weakness, followed by left face and then right face weakness. In the last few weeks, he also complained of bilateral circumoral numbness. During the course of his illness, he lost 25 pounds. Two months prior to the onset of this illness, he had high fever, chills, and night sweats lasting 2 days.

CASE SUMMARY

The 38-year-old man in the video presented with 6 months of multifocal sensory neuropathy/radiculopathy and pain followed by the development of multifocal weakness and multiple cranial neuropathies. The sensory symptoms and signs follow a peripheral or cranial nerve distribution, and his weakness is of a lower motor neuron type. The neurophysiologic studies revealed evidence for a sensory motor peripheral neuropathy in a patchy distribution consistent with mononeuritis multiplex.

The differential diagnosis for multifocal radiculopathies and peripheral and cranial neuropathies (including bilateral facial neuropathies as with the current patient) would lead to a suspicion for a variety of chronic inflammatory or infiltrating conditions. Infectious diseases include Lyme disease, syphilis, cryptococcal meningitis, tuberculous meningitis, and leprosy. In addition, autoimmune inflammatory conditions known to cause mononeuritis multiplex include neurosarcoidosis, polyarteritis nodosa, and other connective tissue diseases and vasculitides. The spectrum of malignancy with carcinomatous meningitis can be one of the more difficult diagnoses to establish with certainty. Cerebrospinal fluid studies have notoriously limited sensitivity and require, in many patients, multiple samplings with high-volume spinal fluid.

Patients with an immune-mediated chronic inflammatory polyradiculoneuropathy tend not to have such a patchy multifocal stuttering course; rather, they have a clinical picture of more symmetric and steadily progressive sensory and motor dysfunction. Patients who have classical aggressive carcinomatous meningitis will typically have a low glucose in cerebrospinal fluid (although the other conditions listed previously will often also be associated with a low glucose), and the CSF cytology can make the diagnosis in many patients. The differential diagnosis for a polyradiculoneuropathy includes diabetes, vasculitic neuropathies, neurosarcoidosis, multiple myeloma, and immune-mediated disorders. Neuroimaging studies showed little in the way of meningeal enhancement.

The initial spinal fluid studies were abnormal, showing an elevated protein, a mild lymphocytic pleocytosis, and a normal or marginal glucose. Initial cytology evaluations on CSF were normal. Because of the patient's progressive clinical course, he underwent a more extensive diagnostic evaluation including body CT scan, which revealed widespread adenopathy. Lymph node biopsy was then diagnostic for B-cell lymphoma.

His management has included systemic chemotherapy with cyclophosphamide, adriamycin, and prednisone. The use of vincristine is problematic given the presence of underlying peripheral neuropathy/radiculopathy and the concerns of superimposed neurotoxicity.

As the blood–brain barrier serves to limit access to systemic drugs for treatment of malignancy, it is not uncommon for central nervous system metastases to be more resistant to systemic therapy. For that reason, radiation therapy and intrathecal chemotherapy are often necessary for management of progressive meningeal disease. This patient responded favorably to systemic chemotherapy for several months. Systemic recurrence has led to alternative therapy, currently stem cell transplantation.

■ **SELECTED REFERENCES**

Biller J, ed. *Practical neurology,* 2nd ed. Philadelphia: Lippincott Williams & Wilkins, 2002.
Posner JB. *Neurologic complications of cancer.* Philadelphia: FA Davis Co, 1995.
Roos KL. Carcinomatous meningitis. In: *Meningitis (100 maxims in neurology).* New York: Oxford University
     Press, 1996:182–198.

■ **SEE QUESTIONS: 137, 151, 154, 155, 194, 215**

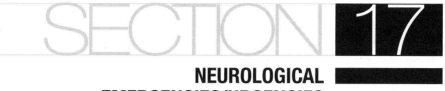

SECTION 17

NEUROLOGICAL EMERGENCIES/URGENCIES

CASE 94

ACUTE CEREBELLAR INFARCTION (PICA) WITH EARLY HYDROCEPHALUS

OBJECTIVES

- To highlight pitfalls in the diagnosis of acute posterior fossa ischemic stroke.
- To review the clinical presentation of acute cerebellar infarction in the PICA territory.
- To review the potential serious consequences of large cerebellar infarctions.
- To discuss management guidelines for these patients.

VIGNETTE

A 41-year-old woman with a history of untreated hyperlipidemia and cigarette smoking was evaluated at an ER three days previously because of new-onset nausea, vomiting, and disequilibrium. Diagnosed to have the flu and depression, she was sent home in a wheelchair. She is now admitted because of occipital headaches and increased unsteadiness.

CASE SUMMARY

Our patient had an acute cerebellar infarction involving the territory of the posterior inferior cerebellar artery (PICA). Fortunately, despite the initial misdiagnosis of depression and the flu, she had a good clinical outcome.

The brainstem, cerebellum, and labyrinths are supplied by the vertebrobasilar arterial system. The areas of the cerebellum supplied by the posterior inferior cerebellar

183

artery (PICA) are extremely variable. There are several different patterns of PICA territory cerebellar infarctions. If the medial branch is affected, involving the vermis and vestibulocerebellum, the clinical findings include prominent vertigo, ataxia, and nystagmus. If the lateral cerebellar hemisphere is involved, patients can have vertigo, gait ataxia, limb dysmetria and ataxia, nausea, vomiting, conjugate or dysconjugate gaze palsies, miosis, and dysarthria.

If the cerebellar infarction is large with a mass effect and compression of the brainstem and fourth ventricle, altered consciousness may develop. Hydrocephalus or herniation may occur. There is also a syndrome of dorsolateral medullary and cerebellar infarction that may be caused by a vertebral artery occlusion or a medial PICA occlusion. Although a PICA occlusion can be the cause of Wallenberg (lateral medullary) syndrome, this syndrome is more often caused by an intracranial vertebral artery occlusion.

Emergency room physicians should have a low threshold for obtaining consultation with a neurologist or neurosurgeon in patients who present with isolated vertigo or with vertigo, imbalance, and nausea, and who also have risk factors for cerebrovascular disease. As many as 25% of patients with cerebrovascular risk factors who present to an emergency room with isolated vertigo, nystagmus, and postural instability have an infarction involving the inferior cerebellum. MRI and MRA are the preferred neuroimaging modalities for evaluating these patients. If MRI is unavailable, CT with fine cuts through the posterior fossa may be used. Careful attention to the status of the brainstem cisterns and fourth ventricle is required.

Patients with cerebellar infarction should be admitted to an intensive care unit or a dedicated stroke unit. In cases of cerebellar infarction with mass effect, when fourth ventricular compression and hydrocephalus are the primary concerns, some neurosurgeons prefer to perform a ventriculostomy; however, this procedure is associated with a risk of upward cerebellar herniation through the free edge of the tentorial incisura. For this reason, other neurosurgeons favor posterior fossa decompressive surgery for these patients.

■ SELECTED REFERENCES

Heros RC. Cerebellar hemorrhage and infarction. *Stroke* 1982;13:106–109.
Hotson JR, Baloh RW. Acute vestibular syndrome. *New Engl J Med* 1998;339:680–685.
Norrving B, Magnusson M, Holtas S. Isolated acute vertigo in the elderly: vestibular or vascular disease? *Acta Neurol Scand* 1995;91:43–48.

■ SEE QUESTIONS: 19, 55, 68, 92, 95, 143, 183

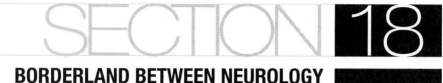

SECTION 18

BORDERLAND BETWEEN NEUROLOGY AND PSYCHIATRY

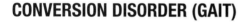

CASE 95

CONVERSION DISORDER (GAIT)

OBJECTIVE

▪ To present an unusual disorder of gait.

VIGNETTE

A 22-year-old woman was admitted with sudden onset of legs buckling under her when she attempted to stand. Her review of systems was normal and her past history was significant for being 2 months postpartum. The patient did admit to feeling overwrought with the stressors of a new baby and her engagement to the baby's father.

CASE SUMMARY

Is her gait dysfunction organic in nature? Despite full strength, normal muscle tone, unremarkable muscle stretch reflexes, normal sensory and cerebellar examination, and lack of involuntary movements, our patient had a bizarre and rather spectacular gait disorder characterized by variability with distraction, slowness and hesitation in walking, and buckling of her knees. Her gait pattern did not resemble a hemiparetic, ataxic, shuffling, steppage or scissor type of gait abnormality, but was rather consistent with a psychogenic disorder of gait.

Somatoform disorders represent a psychiatric condition because the physical symptoms present in this disorder cannot be fully accounted for by a medical disorder, substance use, or another mental disorder. Specific somatoform disorders include

(i) somatization disorder, (ii) conversion disorder, (iii) pain disorder, (iv) hypochondriasis, and (v) body dysmorphic disorder. As stated in the *Diagnostic and Statistical Manual of Mental Disorders,* fourth edition *(DSM-IV)*, conversion disorder involves symptoms or deficits affecting voluntary motor or sensory function that suggest a neurological or other general medical condition.

Gait disorders are very common in the very old and in the very young. Psychogenic gait disorders can take many forms including hemiparetic, paraparetic, and ataxic disorders; dystonic abnormalities; trembling; or, as in our patient, a rather striking buckling of knees.

■ SELECTED REFERENCES

Biller J, ed. *Practical neurology,* 2nd ed. Philadelphia: Lippincott Williams & Wilkins, 2002.
Lemperet T, Brandt T, Dieterich M, et al. How to identify psychogenic disorders of stance and gait. *J Neurol* 1991;238:140–146.

■ SEE QUESTION: 252

CASE 96

CONVERSION DISORDER (SPEECH)

OBJECTIVES

■ To describe the somatoform disorders.
■ To demonstrate an unusual presentation of conversion disorder.
■ To distinguish somatization from factitious disorder and malingering.

VIGNETTE

One month after clipping of an unruptured basilar tip aneurysm, this 43-year-old woman, recently divorced, experienced difficulty producing speech. She has had recent hospitalizations because of unexplained abdominal pain, chest pains, and syncope.

CASE SUMMARY

Six weeks following clipping of an asymptomatic, unruptured, basilar tip aneurysm, our patient began to experience changes in her speech. At first, she was unable to speak at all. This improved, although she then had more trouble generating speech fluently. She also reported having trouble remembering "sequential things." By that she meant she must read instructions a number of times, such as those for getting to our clinic. She had trouble with recipes as well. Her mood was described as pretty good, and she denied any sense of sadness or dysphoria. She did not seem particularly disturbed or upset by the idea that her speech problem might become chronic and prevent her return to work. Postop MRI of the brain and catheter cerebral angiogram showed the basilar tip aneurysm clip, but they were otherwise unremarkable. Ears, nose, and throat (ENT) evaluation showed inconsistent glottal closure with laryngeal tremors.

There were some marked social stressors in our patient's recent past. In addition to her surgery, her husband apparently abruptly left her without warning after 24 years of marriage. He left her for another woman whom she did not know. She denied other prior stressors including financial pressures or health problems in her family or children. She denied any previous problems at work with her colleagues. She reportedly liked her work. She denied any symptoms of obsessive-compulsive disorder, panic disorder, generalized anxiety disorder, schizophrenic disorder, bipolar disorder, or posttraumatic stress disorder.

Examination revealed an awake, alert, and well-oriented woman who provided her own history. She was casually dressed, neatly groomed, and appeared her stated age. Her speech was marked by a kind of stutter on the initial clause of a sentence. Upon beginning a phrase, her eyes rolled closed and her neck torqued (sometimes to the right and sometimes to the left). She squinted as well and occasionally experienced a whole-body jerk. Her mood appeared to be quite euthymic and she smiled or laughed frequently, including during descriptions of traumatic events such as her husband leaving her. Assessment of effort with forced-choice recognition memory was unremarkable. Her thoughts in conversation were logical, sequential, and goal oriented. Her fund of general knowledge was high average and estimated intellectual endowment was average/high average based on word pronunciation.

Her digit span was normal forward and borderline backward. She had difficulty sequencing randomly arranged numbers and letters. Visual motor scanning speed was quite slow, with continued impairment given the added requirements of mental set alteration; performance did improve somewhat. Abstract verbal reasoning with similarities was average. She solved an ambiguous and novel problem with relatively little error or perseveration.

Short-term recall of oral narrative was normal, but there was forgetting over time and mildly impaired long-term retrieval. By contrast, she learned a 15-word list normally with rehearsal with insignificant forgetting over time and normal long-term retrieval and recognition. Short- and long-term recall of geometric figures were both normal, although there was slight forgetting over time.

Despite the speech abnormality, letter fluency was normal, as was confrontation naming. She could write well to dictation, but her writing was not particularly fluent and she wrote with great pressure on the pencil. Constructional praxis in assembling blocks to match a template was average to normal on the nondominant left. Specifically, her grip strength was 20 kg/in^2 on the right hand, which was somewhat inconsistent with the pressure she was applying with her pencil and to hand squeeze. Limb praxis appeared to be essentially normal.

The Minnesota Multiphasic Personality Inventory, MMPI-2, was administered, but the profile was invalid from overly positive self-presentation. That said, there were no obvious indications of depression. The clinical scales themselves were a 1-3 profile, which was associated with individuals who commonly convert psychological distress into somatic complaints. The remainder of the neurological examination was unremarkable.

In summary, we felt that our patient had a rather unusual and inconsistent speech pattern that appeared more functional than neurological. She did not have an aphasic syndrome. We also felt that there was a temporal relationship with relevant psychological stressors and an unconscious motivation for her symptoms. In other words, we felt that her speech problem was not intentional or under voluntary control (as in factitious disorder or malingering). Although the MMPI itself was invalid, given what appeared to be an overly positive self-presentation, there were some indications of a somatoform personality constellation. Similarly, there was evidence of *la belle indifférence* regarding her abnormalities. In addition, there was a mild psychomotor slowing of doubtful significance.

Somatoform disorders represent a psychiatric condition because the physical symptoms present in this disorder cannot be fully accounted for by a medical disorder, substance use, or another mental disorder. Specific somatoform disorders include (i) somatization disorder, (ii) conversion disorder, (iii) pain disorder, (iv) hypochondriasis, and (v) body dysmorphic disorder. As stated in the *Diagnostic and Statistical Manual of Mental Disorders,* fourth edition *(DSM-IV),* conversion disorder involves symptoms or deficits affecting voluntary motor or sensory function that suggest a neurological or other general medical condition.

Yet, following a thorough evaluation, the loss of function is not accounted for by a neurological condition, medical illness, or culturally expected behavioral response. Common conversion symptoms include blindness, diplopia, pseudoseizures, paralysis, anesthesia, midline hemihypalgesia often associated with ipsilateral visual and hearing loss, unresponsiveness, amnesia, aphonia, and mutism. Medication approaches are rarely successful for those patients with conversion disorder. Symptoms often resolve spontaneously.

The patient was reassured that her symptoms were very real although not due to an underlying neurological or other organic disorder. She was subsequently referred to psychiatry for further evaluation and management.

■ SELECTED REFERENCES

American Psychiatric Association. Somatoform disorders. In: *Diagnostic and statistical manual of mental disorders,* 4th ed. Washington, DC: APA Press, 1994:452–457.

Boffeli TJ, Guze SB. The simulation of neurologic disease. *Psychiatric Clin North Am* 1992;15(Jun):301–310.

Fink P, Sorensen L, Engberg M. Somatization in primary care. Prevalence, health care utilization, and general practitioner recognition. Psychosomatics 1999;40(Jul-Aug):330–338.

■ SEE QUESTION: 252

CASE 97

CONVERSION DISORDER (MEIGE SYNDROME)

OBJECTIVES

▧ To demonstrate an unusual presentation of conversion disorder.
▧ To briefly discuss characteristics of idiopathic cranial dystonia and spasmodic dysphonia.

VIGNETTE

A 58-year-old woman has had abnormal movements of the head, neck, and upper extremities since 1998. These episodes began after bumping her back into some bakery shelving at her job. Since then, she has had spasms of both eyes, face, neck, and upper extremities. She is also having breathing difficulties and visual problems because her eyes are shut during these spells.

CASE SUMMARY

Our patient began to have facial grimacing, face turn, neck flexion, and other abnormal posturing of the body soon after an episode of bumping her back into some bakery shelving at her job. Diagnoses of cranial dystonia (Meige syndrome), spasmodic dysphonia, or conversion reaction were entertained by different neurology consultants at different times. MRI of the brain was unremarkable. MRI of the cervical spine showed moderate neural canal stenosis at C5-6. EMG activity of the neck musculature was quiet despite being measured with a dystonic burst of activity. The blink reflex was unremarkable.

Botox injections into the sternocleidomastoid, platysmas, left splenius capitis, medial and lateral lids, lateral canthus, and corrugators did not provide satisfactory relief. Pharmacologic treatment with baclofen, klonopin, gapapentin, propranolol, benzodiazepines, and a variety of antidepressants was unsatisfactory. Investigations for the DYT1GAG deletion was negative. Glutamic acid decarboxylase antibody was less than 1 U/mL (reference range 0.00 to 1.45). Slit lamp examination was unremarkable. Serum copper and ceruloplasmin levels were normal. Thyroid function tests were normal.

Our patient was married and had three children. She did not smoke or consume alcohol. She acknowledged neurovegetative signs of depression, but did not report any suicidal ideations. She was not receiving any neuroleptic drugs. She had a difficult childhood in that her father was physically abusive of his wife as well as both daughters. He also had a significant drinking problem. She apparently had gone through great emotional turmoil related to the death of her father (prostate cancer) and stated that her father had treated her in a very mean way all of her life and that she had very negative feelings toward him. She was at her father's bedside at her father's death. She described her mother as "very controlling."

On examination, she looked older than her stated age. Her voice was somewhat weak and strained, but did not have the tight quality and glottic breaks of classic spasmodic dysphonia. She intermittently had straightening of the trunk, flexion of the neck, face turn toward the left, and slight head tilt toward the left. This was accompanied by spasmodic movements of the upper chest and deviation of the eyes to the right as compensatory eye movement. There was occasional grimacing of the face and tightening of the platysmae and trapezii. During her examination she tended to place her shoulders forward and tended to extend both arms.

It was notable that on occasions where she was spoken to in a supportive manner, she would be able to engage without any abnormal movements for periods of 30 to 45 seconds. Her oral-facial features did seem to vary and were almost continually present, worsening at times of talking about emotionally distressing topics or during actual examination of her eyes. There was no evidence of delusions, hallucinations, or paranoia. Her thought process was linear and logical. She was open to talking about the stressors. Visual acuity was 20/30 in the right eye with correction. Visual acuity in the left eye was 20/40 with correction. Confrontation visual fields were full.

There was a small exophoria at distance that increased at near. The range of eye movements was full. Horizontal and vertical pursuit was jerky. Saccades were normal. Pupils were 5 mm in diameter and had normal reactions. There was no relative afferent pupillary defect. Funduscopy showed normal appearance of the disc, maculae, vessels, and periphery. There was no sign of exophthalmos. Examination of the lids showed no ptosis or blepharospasm. There was no apraxia of lid opening. Jaw jerk was unremarkable. Larynx and hypopharynx showed that both vocal cords were mobile. The remainder of the neurological and general physical examinations were unremarkable.

In summary, our patient had a rather unusual constellation of spasmodic movements of the oral-facial area as well as upper chest, and no evidence of blepharospasm or spasmodic dysphonia. Oromandibular dystonia with blepharospasm, also known as Meige syndrome or Brueghel syndrome, is a rare form of adult-onset cranial dystonia characterized by intense and involuntary spasms of the orbicularis oculi (blepharospasm) and of the lower facial or oromandibular muscles. Women are more affected than men. Its most common and disabling manifestation is blepharospasm. Oromandibular dystonia is the second most common manifestation. The disorder may spread beyond the facial and nuchal musculature to involve one or both arms or the trunk. Most cases are idiopathic or primary.

Secondary Meige syndrome has been reported in association with the chronic administration of neuroleptics, levodopa, or other drugs; cerebellopontine angle meningiomas; and other focal intracranial lesions. It has been postulated that dopamine plays a predominant role in the pathophysiology of Meige syndrome. Spasmodic dysphonia refers to a segmental, and usually nonprogressive, action dystonia characterized by dystonic spasms of the laryngeal muscles, in particular the adductors. Three subtypes of spasmodic dysphonia have been reported: adductor, abductor, and mixed. Extensive neurological evaluation performed in our patient failed to find any organic etiology, and clearly she had psychological themes that cause her a significant level of despair. A diagnosis of conversion disorder was made.

As stated in the *Diagnostic and Statistical Manual of Mental Disorders,* fourth edition *(DSM-IV),* conversion disorder involves symptoms or deficits affecting voluntary motor or sensory function that suggest a neurological or other general medical condition, usually in the context of a severe stressor. Yet, following a thorough evaluation, the loss of function is not accounted for by a neurological condition, medical illness, or culturally expected behavioral response.

Common conversion symptoms include blindness, diplopia, pseudoseizures, hemiparesis, paraparesis, monoparesis, incoordination, anesthesia, midline hemihypalgesia often associated with ipsilateral visual and hearing loss, unresponsiveness, amnesia, aphonia, mutism, bizarre gait disturbances (astasia-abasia), and movement disorders. Conversion disorders can imitate the entire spectrum of movement disorders including dystonia.

■ SELECTED REFERENCES

American Psychiatric Association: Somatoform disorders. In: *Diagnostic and statistical manual of mental disorders,* 4th ed. Washington, DC: APA Press, 1994:452–457.

Boffeli TJ, Guze SB. The simulation of neurologic disease. *Psychiatric Clin North Am* 1992;15(Jun):301–310.

Cannito MP, Johnson JP. Spastic dysphonia: a continuum disorder. *J Commun Disord* 1981;14:215–233.

Tolosa E, Marti MJ. Blepharospasm-oromandibular dystonia syndrome (Meige's syndrome): clinical aspects. *Adv Neurol* 1988;49:73–84.

■ SEE QUESTION: 252

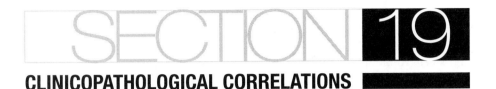

SECTION 19

CLINICOPATHOLOGICAL CORRELATIONS

CASE 98

ISOLATED CNS ANGIITIS

OBJECTIVES

- To review the basic pathophysiology of the vasculitides.
- To review the clinical characteristics of primary central nervous system (CNS) vasculitis.
- To discuss ancillary diagnostic tests in primary CNS vasculitis.
- To review management principles in primary CNS vasculitis.

VIGNETTE

A 30-year-old man had protracted and severe headaches that he attributed to possible migraines. He also had binocular horizontal diplopia, worse when looking to the right. He also had some numbness below the right eyelid that progressed to involve the right side of his skull.

He had numerous investigations including MRIs, MRAs, MRVs, and a cerebral angiogram. MRI showed increased T2 signal on the right cerebellar hemisphere. He was initially thought to have a brain tumor and was seen by a neurosurgeon who disagreed with the diagnosis.

Subsequent investigations suggested the possibility of a cerebellar venous thrombosis with compromised right cerebellar hemispheric venous drainage on a cerebral arteriogram performed in June 2001. There was also a partial thrombosis of one of the right occipital veins draining into the right transverse sinus. A lumbar puncture showed 18 white blood cells, protein of 46, and glucose of 62. There was some elevation of the IgG index and albumin index. The patient was started on warfarin.

Previous attempts to discontinue warfarin were associated with the reappearance of his headaches.

His symptoms have waxed and waned and he had another hospitalization because of frequent vomiting and numbness on the right side of the forehead and right lower lid. He also had some dizziness and ringing in both ears. On November 2, 2001, he was admitted to the hospital because of severe right occipital headaches. His international normalized ratio (INR) on admission was 1.65. Neuroimaging studies obtained during that hospitalization are shown. One day after admission, the patient was taken to the operating room and had a left suboccipital craniotomy.

CASE SUMMARY

Vascular injury is the central pathology in the vasculitides, and the mechanisms of injury are diverse. Vasculitis is characterized by blood vessel inflammation and necrosis. Four basic types of immunopathogenetic mechanisms have been accepted: (i) anaphylactic, (ii) cytotoxic/cell activating, (iii) immune complex, and (iv) cell mediated. Injury can also occur by other pathways including direct cytokine-mediated, direct neutrophil involvement, genetically mediated, direct infectious, or environmental/chemical injury. More than one mechanism is likely to be involved in a particular vasculitis.

The diagnosis of vasculitis is often inferential, based on clinical presentation, presence of multisystem organ involvement, and abnormal serologic tests. Cerebral vasculitis should be considered when the stroke is recurrent, associated with encephalopathic changes, or accompanied by fever, weight loss, fatigue, arthralgias, myalgias, palpable purpura or other skin lesions, renal disease, multifocal neurological signs, anemia, hematuria, or elevated erythrocyte sedimentation rate (ESR).

Primary CNS vasculitis is a rare noninfectious granulomatous, necrotizing angiopathy of unknown cause. Primary CNS vasculitis is characterized by predominant or exclusive involvement of the CNS. Usual symptoms include headaches and mental status changes. Symptoms of predominant small vessel involvement may present as a mass lesion or as a multifocal encephalopathy. Small vessel strokes may occur over weeks to many months. Intracranial hemorrhage is a rare complication of primary CNS vasculitis.

The ESR is usually normal or minimally elevated. Other acute phase reactants are characteristically normal. CSF abnormalities include increased protein values, normal glucose level, and a discrete lymphocytic pleocytosis. Contrast-enhanced MRI studies are abnormal in over 90% of cases. Arteriography may show segmental arterial narrowing, vascular occlusions, peripheral aneurysms, vascular shifts, and avascular areas, or may be entirely unremarkable. Brain leptomeningeal biopsy is essential for diagnosis. Due to the focal nature of the vasculitis, a negative biopsy result does not exclude the diagnosis of primary CNS vasculitis. Management consists of long-term treatment with corticosteroids with the addition of cyclophosphamide in progressive or steroid-resistant cases. Pulse cyclophosphamide has been successfully used in the treatment of primary CNS vasculitis in children.

■ SELECTED REFERENCES

Biller J, Adams HP. Non-infectious granulomatous angiitis of the central nervous system. In: Toole JF, ed. *Handbook of clinical neurology.* Amsterdam: Elsevier Science, 1987:387–400.

Biller J, Loftus CM, Moore SA, et al. Isolated central nervous system angiitis first presenting as spontaneous intracranial hemorrhage. *Neurosurgery* 1987;20:310–315.

■ SEE QUESTIONS: 67, 68, 71, 104, 188, 216, 217

CASE 99

CEREBROTENDINOUS XANTHOMATOSIS

OBJECTIVES

- To review the main neurological features of cerebrotendinous xanthomatosis (CTX).
- To discuss the clinical course and progression of CTX.
- To review diagnostic criteria for CTX.
- To discuss management strategies for CTX.

VIGNETTE

A 64-year-old woman was seen 6 years previously because of several years of progressive gait difficulties. This difficulty has progressed to the point where she had to use a cane for ambulating and recently has been confined to a wheelchair. She had a history of bilateral cataract surgery in her early thirties and "lumps" in both Achilles tendons.

CASE SUMMARY

Our patient presented with a 2-year history of progressive ataxia and memory troubles. She had previously undergone surgery for bilateral cataracts that she developed in her 30s. On neurological examination, she had inappropriate jocularity, mild dysarthria, muscle stretch hyperreflexia, bilateral Babinski signs, mild intention tremor, dysdiadochokinesis, a wide-base unstable gait that required the assistance of a cane, and inability to perform tandem walking. Neuropsychological testing showed widespread neurocognitive deficits with poor attention and concentration, dyscalculia, and impaired memory.

Her serum cholestanol level was elevated at 1.60 mg/dL (normal 0.2 $\pm$ 0.2 mg/dL). Her serum methylmalonic acid, serum B_{12} level, vitamin E levels, and genetic testing for spinocerebellar ataxias were all normal. Cultured fibroblasts were checked for 27-sterol hydroxylase deficiency. Treatment was initiated with chenodeocycholic acid (CDCA). She initially experienced some mild improvement over the next year, but this was followed by progressive neurological deterioration with increasing ataxia, further sensory changes on her limbs, urinary incontinence, and a mild decline on repeat neuropsychological testing. Nerve conduction studies (NCVs) were consistent with a demyelinating neuropathy of the lower extremities.

MRI of the brain was remarkable for increased T2 and FLAIR signal abnormalities along the corticospinal tracts in the periventricular and subcortical white matter of both cerebral hemispheres, posterior limb of the internal capsules, cerebral peduncles, and pons. MRI of the spinal cord was normal. MRS testing in the area of the basal ganglia showed a decreased *N*-acetylaspartate peak and an increased peak of 0.9 to 1.5 over the left basal ganglia that was amino acids versus lipids. MRS of the right occipital region was normal. She then became wheelchair bound and incontinent of urine and feces. Her examination also included decreased vibration and position sense in both feet. It was decided to add atorvastatin along with CDCA in an attempt to prevent further neurological deficits.

Cerebrotendinous xanthomatosis (CTX, Van Bogaert's disease) is a rare autosomal recessive disorder of bile acid synthesis caused by a defect of the mitochondrial enzyme sterol 27-hydroxylase. The disorder is characterized by an accumulation of cholestanol and cholesterin in various tissues. It typically presents as a slowly progressive ataxia in conjunction with tendinous xanthomas. Pyramidal and cerebellar manifestations along with dementia are the predominant neurological manifestations. Various other neurological manifestations have been described including seizures, psychosis, parkinsonism, chronic myelopathy, and peripheral neuropathy.

The xanthomas may also be seen in the quadriceps, triceps, and fingers in addition to the Achilles tendons, or they may be absent. Ophthalmologic findings other than cataracts can be seen including pallor of the optic discs and signs of premature retinal aging. Elevated serum cholestanol and urine bile acid glucuronides help to confirm the diagnosis. The primary treatment of CTX is with the oral administration of chenodeoxycholic acid (CDCA). HMG-CoA reductase inhibitors have also been used.

■ SELECTED REFERENCES

Burnett JR, Moses EA, Croft KD, et al. Clinical and biochemical features, molecular diagnosis and long term management of a case of cerebrotendinous xanthomatosis. *Clinica Chemica Acta* 2001;306(Apr):63–69.

Chen W, Kubota S, Teramoto T, et al. Genetic analysis enables definite and rapid diagnosis of cerebrotendinous xanthomatosis. *Neurology* 1998;51:865–867.

Kuriyama M, Tokimura Y, Fujiyama J, et al. Treatment of cerebrotendinous xanthomatosis: effects of chenodeoxycholic acid, pravastatin, and combined use. *J Neurol Sci* 1994;125(1):22–28.

Van Bogaert L, et al. Une forme cérébrale de la cholestérinose généralise. Paris: Mason et Cie, 1937.

■ SEE QUESTIONS: 27, 251

CASE 100

POLYMYOSITIS/MYASTHENIA GRAVIS

OBJECTIVES

- To identify the principal causes of chronic progressive bulbar weakness.
- To demonstrate the value of clinical and laboratory data to distinguish myasthenia gravis from myositis.
- To outline acute and chronic treatment strategies for immune-mediated neuromuscular disorders.

VIGNETTE

Two years ago, this 53-year-old woman had a left middle cerebral artery territory embolic infarction associated with atrial fibrillation/flutter. She was status post catheter ablation a week prior to her stroke. She was treated with Coumadin and had a good recovery. She then had a maze atrial procedure and Coumadin was discontinued.

She now complains of progressive swallowing difficulties and increased progressive weakness, mostly in the proximal aspect of her extremities. She has also had troubles lifting objects over her head and brushing her hair. She furthermore noticed that she was unable to rise from a chair and had muscle pains and weakness when trying to climb stairs.

CASE SUMMARY

The patient presents with new-onset progressive and severe neuromuscular weakness including dysphagia and dyspnea.

The first priority in a patient complaining of difficulty with speech, swallowing, and breathing is always to make certain that their vital neuromuscular functions are secure. If the patient is overtly aspirating or choking frequently with meals or losing weight precipitously, it is best to admit him or her on an urgent basis to assess the swallowing more thoroughly and adjust the PO intake appropriately. Similarly, if there is any question about pulmonary status, it is best to deal with that on an urgent basis before pursuing further diagnostic tests.

A vigorous cough will provide a rough estimate to the patient's pulmonary function; taking a deep breath and then counting out loud is an excellent method of estimating forced vital capacity. If the person can count to 10 on one breath, their forced vital capacity is 1 liter. If they can count to 25 on one breath, then they have 2 liters of forced vital capacity. In general, patients with neuromuscular or respiratory failure who are acutely deteriorating should be considered as severe enough to warrant intubation and mechanical ventilation when forced vital capacity drops below 1 liter (or 15 mL/kg).

In the current patient, there is evidence of proximal weakness as well as bulbar weakness. Proximal symmetrical weakness is typical for a myopathy. However, oropharyngeal musculature can be affected in a variety of myopathies including inflammatory and immune-mediated conditions such as dermatomyositis, polymyositis, and inclusion body myositis. Patients over age 50 who have dermatomyositis have the strongest association with malignancy (present in 25% of patients), whereas those patients under age 50 and those with polymyositis have a far lower likelihood of associated cancer. At times the degree of oropharyngeal weakness can be severe. In some patients, it is the predominant site of involvement. These patients' creatine kinase is elevated, supporting the diagnosis of an inflammatory myopathy. Elevation of creatine kinase and also aldolase in the current patient supports the diagnosis of a myopathy.

Neurophysiological studies can be a powerful tool in defining a neuromuscular condition. This patient had normal nerve conduction studies. There was no decrement to 2-Hz repetitive stimulation. A decremental response is typically evidence for a defect of neuromuscular transmission. However, only 50% of patients with myasthenia gravis (MG) demonstrate a decremental response to repetitive stimulation. Therefore, a normal study does not rule out the diagnosis of MG. Single-fiber EMG has a 90% sensitivity but has a limited availability. On EMG needle exam, this patient did have fibrillation and small voluntary motor units. The small motor units indicate the presence of a myopathy, whereas the presence of fibrillation indicates an active component, typical for an inflammatory myopathy. EMG will not distinguish between the various types of inflammatory myopathy.

This patient's muscle biopsy demonstrates muscle fiber necrosis and inflammatory infiltrate consistent with polymyositis. Dermatomyositis has distinctive findings on muscle biopsy with perifascicular muscle fiber atrophy and perivascular inflammation.

Additionally, the patient's bulbar weakness is somewhat labile and fluctuates, raising the question of myasthenia gravis. She has acetylcholine receptor antibodies present on serologic testing. False positives with this test are exceedingly rare; in a patient with fluctuating bulbar weakness, the diagnosis of MG should be secure. Patients with one autoimmune neuromuscular disease have an increased chance of having other immune-mediated conditions including other neuromuscular disorders. There is an established association between myositis and myasthenia gravis, and in this case, the patient probably has two different conditions affecting the neuromuscular junction and muscle to account for her severe weakness. Patients with a combination of myasthenia gravis and myositis should be carefully screened for thymoma.

The fact that the patient has severe bulbar weakness and there is a tendency for it to exacerbate over a period of days would suggest sufficient fluctuation and lability to favor myasthenia gravis as the predominant mechanism for her bulbar weakness. Therefore, treatment with cholinesterase inhibitors and immunosuppression would be appropriate. Immunosuppressive drugs used in myasthenia gravis include high-dose long-term corticosteroids, azathioprine, mycophenolate, and cyclosporine. Short-term treatment for patients severely affected or acutely decompensated include plasma exchange and i.v. Ig.

Treatment options for dermatomyositis and polymyositis include high-dose long-term prednisone (three-fourths of the patients respond fairly well, but the response is slow, often taking up to 8 weeks before the patient begins to experience clinical improvement). Methotrexate and i.v. Ig represent alternative immunotherapies. Inclusion body myositis tends to occur in older patient with a more chronic course measured over years with a preponderance of quadriceps, upper arm, and forearm and finger flexor muscle involvement. Such patients can have significant oropharyngeal involvement as well. Inclusion body myositis tends not to respond to immunotherapy.

■ SELECTED REFERENCES

Biller J, ed. *Practical neurology,* 2nd ed. Philadelphia: Lippincott Williams & Wilkins, 2002.
Kissell JT. Misunderstanding, misperceptions and mistakes in the management of the inflammatory myopathies. *Semin Neurol* 2002;22:41–51.

■ SEE QUESTIONS: 11, 17, 73, 74

CASE 101

SUPRANUCLEAR VERTICAL GAZE PALSY

OBJECTIVES

- To demonstrate a supranuclear disorder of ocular motility.
- To discuss differential diagnosis of supranuclear vertical gaze palsy.

VIGNETTE

Early in 2001, this 49-year-old woman began to have vertigo and binocular vertical diplopia. By the fall of 2001, she began to notice difficulty while looking downward and some variable ptosis of the eyelids. She also had some swallowing difficulties. She had no history of falls or cognitive deterioration. There was a history of arterial hypertension and sleep apnea treated with CPAP.

CASE SUMMARY

Early in 2001, our patient began to have vertigo and binocular vertical diplopia. By the fall of 2001, she began to notice difficulty while looking downward and some variable ptosis of the eyelids. She also had some swallowing difficulties. She had no history of falls or cognitive deterioration. There was a history of arterial hypertension and sleep apnea treated with CPAP. On examination, visual acuity on the right eye was 20/40+1 with correction. Pinhole increased acuity to 20/30. The left eye was 20/40 with correction. Pinhole increased acuity to 20/30. Confrontation visual fields were full. The range of eye movements was full, except for limitation of supraduction in the right eye to 30 degrees and in the left to 35 degrees.

In addition, with verbal instruction and volitional saccades, downward movements were limited to about 20 degrees in each eye. Smooth pursuit horizontally was normal, although it was difficult to judge because of decreased velocity of horizontal saccades. Horizontal saccades had normal amplitudes but a moderate decrease in velocity. Vertical saccades had marked decreased velocities, especially downward. Attempted downward saccades were also hypometric. With the doll's eye maneuver, the ranges of horizontal and vertical movements were normal. Bell's testing did not increase in supraduction. Fixation normally suppressed vestibular nystagmus. There was no pathologic nystagmus.

Pupils were 3 mm in diameter and had decreased direct reactions in each eye. However, there was no relative afferent pupillary defect. Funduscopy showed normal appearances of the disc, maculae, vessels, and periphery. Strength of facial muscles was normal. There was no sign of fatigue of the lid levators or lid twitch sign. The patient did not exhibit eyelid apraxia, paucity of eye blinking, any tremor, limb or axial rigidity, myoclonus, or postural instability. She had no oculomasticatory myorhythmia. The remainder of the neurologic examination was unremarkable.

Her vertical gaze paresis was overcome by passive head movements, which activates the oculocephalic reflexes. Hence, our clinical impression was supranuclear vertical gaze palsy. However, there was also slowing of horizontal saccades. The supranuclear vertical gaze palsy brought to mind possible basal ganglia or midbrain abnormalities. The bilateral slowing of horizontal saccades raised the possibility of lower brainstem problems as well. In addition, she had a skew deviation and mild cataracts.

The major control center of vertical gaze is the rostral interstitial nucleus of the medial longitudinal fasciculus (riMLF). The differential diagnosis of a supranuclear vertical gaze paresis includes a myriad of conditions such as progressive supranuclear palsy (PSP), olivopontocerebellar atrophy, ataxia telangiectasia, dentatorubropallidoluysian atrophy, myasthenia gravis, adult onset Niemann-Pick C disease (sea blue histiocytosis syndrome), adult form of hexosaminidase A deficiency (GM2-gangliosidosis type III), Whipple's disease, Huntington's disease, paraneoplastic brainstem encephalitis, Parkinson's disease, idiopathic striatopallidodentate calcifications, autosomal dominant parkinsonism and dementia with pallidonigral degeneration, Hallervorden-Spatz disease, diffuse Lewy body disease, syphilis, and hypothyroidism.

Our patient had a normal MRI. The pons and cerebellum were unremarkable. There was no thinning of the quadrigeminal plate, no rostral midbrain atrophy, and no evidence of decreased signal intensity in the globus pallidus. MRA of the extracranial and intracranial circulation was normal. Chest roentgenogram was unremarkable. On a video esophagogram, there was incomplete relaxation of the cricopharyngeus muscle. The tensilon test was negative. Results of acetylcholine receptor (muscle) binding antibodies was 0.00 nmol/L (less than or equal to 0.02 nmol/L). Serum hexosaminidase A and total level was 23.7 U/L (10.4 to 23.8). Serum TSH and T4 were normal. Serum vitamin B_{12} was unremarkable. LDH and aldolase were normal.

Serum copper was 166 mcg/dL (70 to 180), and serum ceruloplasmin was 55.7 mg/dL (14 to 57). FTA-ABS and HIV serology were unremarkable. The paraneoplastic antibody panel was negative. CSF analysis showed 2 WBCs, a glucose of 61 mg/dL, and a slight protein elevation at 73 mg/dL. She also had a negative CSF Whipple's disease–associated DNA by PCR. Jejunal biopsy showed no evidence of Whipple's disease. Huntington's disease DNA gene testing was unremarkable. There were no mutations observed in the PANK 2 gene (Hallervorden-Spatz syndrome). Biopsy of the left iliac crest showed a normocellular bone marrow with trilineage hematopoiesis, and no evidence of storage disease. The MELAS and MERRF screen was unremarkable.

We suspect she may have an atypical presentation of PSP (Steele-Richardson-Olszewski syndrome). Neuropathological abnormalities in PSP are mainly located in the pallidum, subthalamic nucleus, substantia nigra, pontine tegmentum, striatum, and periaqueductal gray matter. Recent studies suggest that PSP is a recessive disorder due to an alteration of the gene in chromosome 17 coding for the tau protein (tauopathy). A deficient generation of the motor command by midbrain burst neurons seems to be the likely cause of the abnormal vertical saccades in PSP. No drug or surgical procedure has been shown effective in PSP.

■ SELECTED REFERENCES

Albers DS, Augood SJ. New insights into progressive supranuclear palsy. *Trends Neurosci* 2001;24:347–353.

Bhidayasiri R, Riley DE, Somers JT, et al. Pathophysiology of slow vertical saccades in progressive supranuclear palsy. *Neurology* 2001;57:2070–2077.

Brazis PW, Masdeu JC, Biller J. *Localization in clinical neurology,* 4th ed. Philadelphia: Lippincott Williams & Wilkins, 2001.

Friedman DI, Jancovic J, McCrary JA. Neuro-ophthalmic findings in progressive supranuclear palsy. *J Clin Neuro-Ophthalmol* 1992;12:104–109.

■ SEE QUESTIONS: 27, 42

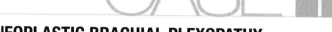

NEOPLASTIC BRACHIAL PLEXOPATHY

OBJECTIVES

- To discuss the anatomy of the brachial plexus.
- To discuss the distinguishing features of a radiation-induced versus a neoplastic plexopathy.

VIGNETTE

A 57-year-old woman with breast carcinoma had right upper extremity weakness.

CASE SUMMARY

This 57-year-old woman was evaluated for weakness of the right arm and hand. She had initially undergone a right mastectomy and chemotherapy for breast cancer. Because of recurrent tumor she had more chemotherapy and had radiation therapy to the right shoulder/axilla. She complained of weakness of the right arm and hand and pain under her right scapula. Examination revealed no evidence of a Horner's syndrome, atrophy of her right forearm, and weakness of multiple muscles of the right upper extremity including the supraspinatus, deltoid, biceps, brachioradialis, triceps, wrist and finger extensors, finger flexors, and multiple intrinsic hand muscles. The weakness of the triceps and wrist extensors was especially severe.

Muscle stretch reflexes in the arms are diffusely hypoactive. A trace triceps reflex was noted on the left but none on the right. Pinprick sensation was diminished on the right thumb, middle finger, and medial forearm. EMG/nerve conduction studies were abnormal with acute denervation changes noted in muscles innervated by multiple nerves and mild abnormalities noted on median and ulnar motor and sensory nerve conductions. This was most indicative of an acute brachial plexopathy. No myokymia was noted. MRI of the right axilla/brachial plexus did demonstrate axillary lymphadenopathy. The patient was diagnosed with a right brachial plexopathy due to metastatic lymphadenopathy.

The brachial plexus is divided into five major components: roots, trunks, divisions, cords, and branches (Fig. 102.1). The five roots are derived from C-5 through T-1. The three trunks are named the upper, middle, and lower trunks. The three trunks separate into three anterior and three posterior divisions. The divisions unite to form three cords named the posterior, lateral, and medial cords. The cords pass through the space of the first rib and clavicle and then give off the major terminal branches or peripheral nerves. Branches of the lateral cord consist of the musculocutaneous nerve and lateral head of the median nerve. Branches of the medial cord consist of the

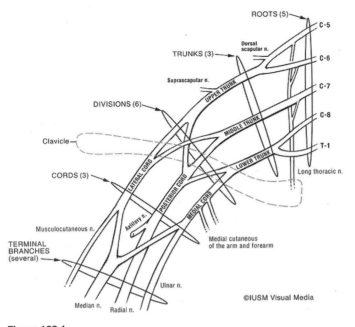

Figure 102.1
Anatomical Drawing of Brachial Plexus

medial anterior thoracic nerve, medial cutaneous nerve of the arm, medial cutaneous nerve of the forearm, ulnar nerve, and median head of the median nerve. Branches of the posterior cord consist of the subscapular nerve, thoracodorsal nerve, axillary nerve, and radial nerve.

Given the relatively complex anatomy of the brachial plexus, it is easy to see that lesions of it can produce a multitude of different signs and symptoms, usually pain, weakness and numbness of various parts of the affected shoulder, arm, and hand. A brachial plexopathy is a well-recognized complication of cancer, especially breast and lung cancer, which are quite common. Many of these patients have received radiation to the axilla or chest to treat their tumors. Distinguishing between a radiation-induced plexopathy and a neoplastic plexopathy is not always easy. Pain occurring in conjunction with the signs and symptoms of the brachial plexopathy would suggest a neoplastic process. Some have suggested that lower trunk lesions occur more frequently with tumors, whereas radiation injuries affect the upper plexus more frequently.

However, this does not appear to be a consistent finding. The presence of a Horner's syndrome is more common in neoplastic processes, whereas lymphedema of the affected arm is more common in radiation injury. Patients with neoplasms tend to have a more aggressive or rapid course of the signs and symptoms (usually over a few months) compared with those with radiation-induced lesions. There is little in the way of electrophysiologic studies to distinguish the two types of brachial plexopathy except that myokymic discharges on needle examination are much more common in radiation-induced plexopathies. Radiologic imaging of the plexus with CT or MRI may show discrete tumors or lymphadenopathy involving the plexus.

■ SELECTED REFERENCES

Brazis PW, Masdeu JC, Biller J, eds. *Localization in clinical neurology*, 4th ed. Philadelphia: Lippincott Williams & Wilkins, 2001.

Harper CM, Thomas JE, Cascino TL, et al. Distinction between neoplastic and radiation-induced brachial plexopathy, with emphasis on the role of EMG. *Neurology* 1989;39:502–506.

Kori SH, Foley KM, Posner JB. Brachial plexus lesions in patients with cancer: 100 cases. *Neurology* 1981;31:45–50.

■ SEE QUESTIONS: 4, 59, 79, 81, 229

REVIEW QUESTIONS AND ANSWERS

1. A 50-year-old man complains of trouble chewing for the past year. He has a history of hypertension, cataract surgery, renal stones, and right bundle branch block on EKG (but no clinical cardiac symptoms). On examination, jaw closure is weak, with 4/5 neck flexion, deltoid, brachioradialis, and quadriceps strength (active movement against gravity and resistance—Medical Research Council 0 to 5/5 scale). No fatigability is found. His hands stiffen with repeated attempts at squeezing the examiner's fingers. Reflexes and sensation are preserved. Mild bilateral eyelid ptosis is noted with normal extraocular movements. What is the most likely clinical diagnosis?

   A. Myasthenia gravis
   B. Myotonic dystrophy
   C. Polymyositis
   D. Myotonia congenita
   E. Amyotrophic lateral sclerosis
   Answer B

2. A 20-year-old woman has a 2-week history of bilateral eyelid ptosis and horizontal diplopia when driving home from work every day. She has no other complaints or past medical history. Her office examination is normal, with no abnormal movements or fatigability of voice, neck, or limbs. However, after 1 minute of sustained upgaze, she develops 2 mm of bilateral asymmetric eyelid ptosis. Which of the following statements is most correct?

   A. She has ocular myasthenia gravis
   B. She has progressive external ophthalmoplegia
   C. Her ocular symptoms may later progress into generalized myasthenia gravis
   D. She has thyroid ophthalmopathy
   E. She may have an internuclear ophthalmoplegia
   Answer C

3. Select the most characteristic clinical feature or differential diagnosis in carpal tunnel syndrome (CTS).

   A. Occurs with greater frequency in men and in the dominant hand
   B. Sensory symptoms can be mimicked by the neurogenic thoracic outlet syndrome
   C. A Tinel's sign has a high specificity as a clinical feature in CTS
   D. An early symptom of CTS is asymmetric nocturnal hand paresthesias
   E. A similar pattern of hand weakness can be seen in a C-7 radiculopathy
   Answer D

4. A clinical condition that could be confused with a retrohumeral radial neuropathy is:

   A. C-8 radiculopathy
   B. Anterior interosseus neuropathy

C. A lesion of the upper trunk of the brachial plexus
D. Posterior interosseus neuropathy
E. C-6 radiculopathy

Answer D

5. The differential diagnosis of a unilateral foot drop would include:

A. S-1 radiculopathy
B. Superficial peroneal mononeuropathy
C. Proximal sciatic mononeuropathy with involvement of the tibial nerve division
D. L-4 radiculopathy
E. Deep peroneal mononeuropathy

Answer E

6. Juvenile absence epilepsy is associated with:

A. Relatively high incidence of absence status
B. Age of onset from 4 to 8 years
C. Generalized tonic-clonic seizures in 40%
D. Generalized 3-Hz-spike wave pattern on EEG
E. Numerous seizures (hundreds) per day

Answer A

7. In juvenile myoclonic epilepsy:

A. Benzodiazepines are contraindicated due to the risk of seizure exacerbation
B. Seizure types include myoclonic jerks and generalized seizures; absence seizures do not occur
C. Treatment is lifelong and seizures recur in virtually all patients after withdrawal of therapy
D. The syndrome is significantly more common in men than in women
E. Patients may be weaned off therapy after the age of 20, provided there has been a seizure-free period of at least 5 years

Answer C

8. Common side effects associated with the use of topiramate in the treatment of epilepsy include all of the following except:

A. Weight loss
B. Hepatotoxicity
C. Elevated intraocular pressure
D. Cognitive dysfunction
E. Increased incidence of renal calculi

Answer B

9. Vagus nerve stimulation therapy for epilepsy is indicated in the following clinical situation:

A. First-line therapy for temporal lobe epilepsy due to mesial temporal sclerosis with documented hippocampal atrophy on MRI

B. Adjunctive therapy for treatment-resistant idiopathic generalized epilepsy

C. Alternative to temporal lobectomy in mesial temporal lobe epilepsy

D. Adjunctive therapy for treatment-resistant focal epilepsy

E. First-line therapy in extratemporal, nonlesional focal epilepsy with secondarily generalized tonic-clonic seizures

Answer D

10. A 30-year-old healthy man presents to the emergency room with a 3- to 4-day history of progressive tingling and numbness in both hands and feet. On examination, he has diffuse 4/5 strength (active movement against gravity and resistance—Medical Research Council 0 to 5/5 scale), distal more than proximal. Muscle stretch reflexes are absent. Sensory examination shows decreased pinprick in both hands and feet and normal position and vibration sense. Which of the following is the most likely diagnosis?

A. Transverse myelitis

B. Guillain-Barré syndrome

C. Polymyositis

D. Amyotrophic lateral sclerosis

E. Myasthenia gravis

Answer B

11. A 30-year-old woman with a history of systemic lupus erythematosus has a 3- to 4-week history of progressively worsening muscle weakness and myalgias. On examination, she has diffuse 4/5 strength (active movement against gravity and resistance—Medical Research Council 0 to 5/5 scale) in both upper and lower extremities, proximal more than distal. Muscle stretch reflexes and sensory examination are normal. Which of the following is the most likely diagnosis?

A. Transverse myelitis

B. Guillain-Barré syndrome

C. Polymyositis

D. Amyotrophic lateral sclerosis

E. Myasthenia gravis

Answer C

12. A 30-year-old woman is seen in the emergency room with a 2-day history of progressively worsening tingling and numbness in both lower extremities. She lost control of her bladder since this morning and also has difficulties moving her legs. On examination, she has diffuse 2/5 strength (active movement with gravity eliminated—Medical Research Council 0 to 5/5 scale). Muscle stretch reflexes are hyperactive and she has bilateral Babinski signs. There is a sensory level to pinprick at T-10. Which of the following is the most likely diagnosis?

A. Transverse myelitis

B. Guillain-Barré syndrome

C. Polymyositis
D. Amyotrophic lateral sclerosis
E. Myasthenia gravis

Answer A

13. A 30-year-old woman is seen in the emergency room because of binocular horizontal diplopia worse on looking to the right. She has also noticed droopy
eyelids in the late hours of the day and admits being "dead tired" by the end of
the day. Neurological examination is normal except for minimal bilateral asymmetric eyelid ptosis and complaints of double vision on right gaze. Which of the
following is the most likely diagnosis?

A. Transverse myelitis
B. Guillain-Barré syndrome
C. Polymyositis
D. Amyotrophic lateral sclerosis
E. Myasthenia gravis

Answer E

14. Following surgery for a ruptured abdominal aortic aneurysm, a 60-year-old
man developed bilateral lower extremity weakness. On examination he has flaccid paraparesis with absent muscle stretch reflexes and no response to plantar
stimulation. Sensory examination shows decreased pinprick sensation with a
T-10 sensory level. Position and vibration sense are preserved. Which of the
following is the most likely diagnosis?

A. Transverse myelitis
B. Guillain-Barré syndrome
C. Brown-Séquard syndrome (hemisection of the spinal cord)
D. Amyotrophic lateral sclerosis
E. Spinal cord infarction

Answer E

15. A 50-year-old man has stiffness and twitching in most of his muscle groups,
progressively getting worse for the last 2 months. On examination he has fasciculations on his right deltoid and right gastrocnemius muscles, with wasting and
weakness of the right hand interossei muscles. Muscle stretch reflexes are bilaterally hyperactive, and he has bilateral Babinski signs. Which of the following is
the most likely diagnosis?

A. Transverse myelitis
B. Guillain-Barré syndrome
C. Polymyositis
D. Amyotrophic lateral sclerosis
E. Myasthenia gravis

Answer D

16. A 30-year-old healthy man recently involved in a motor vehicle accident presents
with neck pain radiating to the right shoulder, lateral aspect of the forearm, right

thumb, and index finger. Neurological examination shows diminished right biceps and brachioradialis reflexes. Which of the following is the most likely diagnosis?

A. Right carpal tunnel syndrome
B. Right C-6 radiculopathy
C. Guillain-Barré syndrome
D. Parsonage-Turner syndrome
E. Cervical myelopathy

Answer B

17. A 30-year-old woman has a 3-month history of numbness in both hands, more so in her right hand. The numbness is mainly nocturnal and on doing manual activities. The numbness fades away on gentle shaking of her hands. She has no neck pain or weakness. She has gained 40 pounds in the last 4 months. On examination, she has decreased pinprick sensation on her right thumb and index finger and a positive Tinel sign at both wrists. Which of the following pair of tests might better explain her clinical problem?

A. Sedimentation rate/ANA titer
B. MRI of cervical spine/CSF analysis
C. MRI of cervical spine/somatosensory evoked potentials
D. Acetylcholine receptor antibodies/chest CT
E. TSH/EMG-NCVs

Answer E

18. Which of the following neurological disorders carries the worst prognosis for survival whether treated or untreated?

A. Transverse myelitis
B. Guillain-Barré syndrome
C. Polymyositis
D. Amyotrophic lateral sclerosis
E. Myasthenia gravis

Answer D

19. The most common symptom of cerebellar infarction is:

A. Vertigo/dizziness
B. Diplopia
C. Paralysis of all volitional movements
D. Convergence retraction nystagmus
E. Head tilt

Answer A

20. Transtentorial herniation may result in infarction of which of the following brain areas?

A. Supramarginal gyrus
B. Superior temporal gyrus

C. Hypothalamus
D. Bilateral inferior frontal gyrus
E. Temporooccipital

Answer E

21. The structure most responsible for the generation of absence seizures is:

A. Hippocampus
B. Hypothalamus
C. Thalamus
D. Temporal lobe
E. Corpus callosum

Answer C

22. Automatisms can occur in which of the following seizure types?

A. Myoclonic
B. Tonic
C. Absence
D. Generalized tonic-clonic
E. Simple partial

Answer C

23. The prevalence of epilepsy in the United States is approximately:

A. 250,000
B. 2.5 million
C. 1 million
D. 10 million
E. 20 million

Answer B

24. Ethosuximide (Zarontin) is used mainly in which of the following seizure types:

A. Generalized tonic-clonic
B. Partial
C. Absence
D. Myoclonic
E. Gelastic

Answer C

25. Complex partial seizures by definition refers to seizures that:

A. Manifest with convulsions
B. Are prolonged
C. Begin in childhood
D. Are associated with an alteration of consciousness
E. Are resistant to medications

Answer D

26. A 5-year-old boy with Down syndrome has had two previous episodes of right facial droop and limp right arm following bouts of crying. The first two episodes resolved within a few hours. His parents brought him in this time because it has lasted more than 4 hours. In the ER he is crying intermittently, has a flattened right nasolabial fold, and pushes you away with the left arm but not the right. What is the most likely diagnosis?

A. Stereotypical behavior typical of Down syndrome
B. Todd's paresis
C. Migraine
D. Moyamoya
E. Brachial plexopathy

Answer D

27. A 9-year-old girl has had progressive difficulty with balance over the past 3 years. She has dysarthria, scoliosis, and mild hearing loss. She has no muscle stretch reflexes and has decreased vibration sense at the toes. An older brother who had similar initial symptoms ended up in a wheelchair and died of a "heart attack" at age 22. What is the most likely diagnosis?

A. Glutaric aciduria
B. Friedreich ataxia
C. Ataxia-telangiectasia
D. Sea-blue histiocytosis
E. MELAS

Answer B

28. Ipsilateral paralysis of adduction of the right eye on volitional gaze with monocular nystagmus of the abducting left eye indicates a lesion of which of the following anatomical structures?

A. Right medial longitudinal fasciculus
B. Left medial longitudinal fasciculus
C. Right central tegmental tract
D. Left central tegmental tract
E. Dentatorubral tract

Answer A

29. Which of the following is the most common cause of ischemic stroke in children?

A. Moyamoya disease
B. Cardiac disease
C. Progeria
D. Kawasaki disease
E. Homocystinuria

Answer B

30. Paradoxical embolization leading to transient ischemic attacks or stroke is a complication of which of the following disorders?

A. Turner syndrome
B. Coarctation of the aorta
C. Rendu-Osler-Weber syndrome
D. Interrupted aortic arch
E. Williams syndrome

Answer C

31. Which of the following organisms infecting the CNS is most common among cardiac transplant patients?

A. *Neisseria meningitidis*
B. *Streptococcus pneumoniae*
C. *Escherichia coli*
D. *Aspergillus fumigatus*
E. *Pseudomonas aeruginosa*

Answer D

32. Which of the following is a significant risk factor for stroke associated with coronary artery bypass graft?

A. Male gender
B. Hypercholesterolemia
C. Left ventricular hypertrophy
D. Aortic arch atherosclerosis
E. Hyperhomocysteinemia

Answer D

33. Facio-pharyngo-laryngo-glosso-masticatory supranuclear palsy results from bilateral infarction of which of the following structures?

A. Brainstem tegmentum
B. Central tegmental tract
C. Operculae and insula
D. Medial temporooccipital region
E. Parietooccipital region

Answer C

34. Anosognosia for cortical blindness results from lesions of which of the following regions:

A. Bilateral parietooccipital
B. Bilateral medial temporooccipital
C. Basal forebrain
D. Bioccipital (area 17)
E. Diagonal band of Broca

Answer D

35. The pain and temperature component of the trigeminal lemniscus originates from which of the following anatomical structures?

A. Pars rostralis
B. Pars interpolaris
C. Pars caudalis
D. Aberrant fibers of Dejerine
E. Nucleus solitarius

Answer C

36. Which of the following pathways decussate at the medullocervical junction?

A. Conjugate horizontal gaze system
B. Dorsal tegmental decussation of Meynert
C. Corticobulbar axons to nuclei of cranial nerves III and IV
D. Corticobulbar axons to nuclei of cranial nerves V, VI, and VII
E. Pyramidal tract

Answer E

37. When the head of an infant is slowly turned to one side, the normal response is characterized by which of the following features?

A. Extension of the arm and leg on the side to which the head is turned
B. Flexion of the arm and leg on the side to which the head is turned
C. Flexion of both arms and legs
D. Extension and pronation of both arms
E. Extension of both legs

Answer A

38. Ipsilateral loss of the corneal reflex in the Wallenberg lateral medullary syndrome results from involvement of which of the following anatomical structures?

A. Descending sympathetic tract
B. Spinal trigeminal nucleus
C. Lateral spinothalamic tract
D. Central tegmental tract
E. Reticular substance

Answer B

39. Which of the following sensory modalities is mediated by both dorsal and ventral column pathways?

A. Pain
B. Temperature
C. Touch
D. Vibration
E. Position

Answer C

40. A 63-year-old woman with Parkinson's disease experiences severe dystonic dyskinesia 2.5 hours later, toward the end of the effect of her levodopa (Sinemet

25/100, 1 tablet po qid). Her dyskinesia lasts for up to 2 hours. What would be the most appropriate management plan for this patient?

A. Decrease the frequency of levodopa to 100 mg po tid
B. Increase the frequency of levodopa to 5 times per day
C. Increase the individual doses of levodopa to 150 mg po qid
D. Add and optimize a dopamine agonist
E. Add selegiline

Answer D

41. A 78-year-old man with an 18-year history of Parkinson's disease is brought to the emergency department with visual hallucinations and agitation. He takes a combination of several antiparkinsonian medications including amantadine, levodopa, selegiline, and pergolide. He does not take other medications with potential to cause encephalopathy. What would be the most appropriate medication adjustment to control hallucinations and agitation in this patient?

A. Add risperidone to control the hallucinations and agitation
B. Stepwise discontinuation of antiparkinsonian medications as needed (i.e., (i) amantadine, (ii) selegiline, (iii) pergolide, (iv) levodopa)
C. Add olanzapine and discontinue amantadine, selegiline, and pergolide
D. Stop all the antiparkinsonian medications
E. Add an acetylcholinesterase inhibitor and olanzapine

Answer B

42. A 60-year-old woman with a 2-year history of speech difficulties, stiffness, and frequent falls comes to the clinic for evaluation. On examination she had evidence of axial rigidity, slow soft speech, a markedly diminished eye blinking rate with normal pursuit eye movements, and a tendency to have motor perseveration. There's also slight tremulousness of the right hand during the finger-to-nose task. Which of the following is the most likely diagnosis?

A. Progressive supranuclear palsy (PSP)
B. Parkinson's disease (PD)
C. Corticobasal degeneration (CBD)
D. Multiple system atrophy (MSA)
E. Dementia with Lewy bodies (DLB)

Answer A

43. A 65-year-old hypertensive woman with a history of diabetes and hyperlipidemia develops abrupt, painless, monocular visual loss of her right eye. On examination, visual acuity is 20/50 OD and 20/20 OS. The superior aspect of her right optic nerve head is edematous. Visual fields show an inferior altitudinal defect. Which of the following is the most likely diagnosis?

A. Posterior ischemic optic neuropathy
B. Central retinal artery occlusion
C. Branch retinal artery occlusion

D. Anterior ischemic optic neuropathy

E. Central retinal vein occlusion

Answer D

44. Which of the following neurological disorders has been associated with the use of sildenafil (Viagra)?

A. Cluster headaches

B. Tics

C. Peripheral neuropathy

D. Myopathy

E. Anterior ischemic optic neuropathy

Answer E

45. Which of the following is the accepted time for treating irreversible retinal ischemia?

A. 180 minutes

B. 24 hours

C. 48 hours

D. 72 hours

E. 96 hours

Answer A

46. Typically, most strokes in patients with Fabry disease (alpha-galactosidase-A deficiency) are characterized by which of the following?

A. Hemorrhagic nature

B. Predominant involvement of the carotid circulation

C. Predominant involvement of the vertebrobasilar circulation

D. Predominant involvement of the spinal cord

E. Predominantly in women

Answer C

47. Which of the following vessels supplies the midbrain, thalamus, and medial aspect of the temporal lobes and occipital lobes?

A. Anterior cerebral artery

B. Middle cerebral artery

C. Posterior cerebral artery

D. Posterior communicating artery

E. Anterior choroidal artery

Answer C

48. Which of the following vessels supplies anatomical structures on both sides of the midline?

A. Anterior cerebral artery

B. Middle cerebral artery

C. Posterior cerebral artery

D. Central artery of Percheron

E. Recurrent artery of Heubner

Answer D

49. A preserved level of consciousness in patients with the locked-in syndrome indicates sparing of which of the following anatomical structures?

A. Pontine tegmentum

B. Paramedian pontine reticular formation (PPRF)

C. Medial longitudinal fasciculus (MLF)

D. Central tegmental tract

E. Midbrain tectum

Answer A

50. Atherosclerotic occlusive disease of the vertebrobasilar circulation affects predominantly which of the following vessels?

A. Distal third of the basilar artery

B. Vertebral artery siphon (V3)

C. Distal intracranial vertebral arteries and proximal and middle segment of basilar artery

D. Distal subclavian arteries

E. Posterior inferior cerebellar arteries

Answer C

51. Ipsilateral conjugate gaze palsy and internuclear ophthalmoplegia result from a lesion simultaneously involving which of the following anatomical structures?

A. Paramedian pontine reticular formation (PPRF) and medial longitudinal fasciculus (MLF)

B. Sixth nerve fascicle and medial longitudinal fasciculus (MLF)

C. Sixth nerve fascicle and rostral interstitial nucleus of the medial longitudinal fasciculus (riMLF)

D. Mollaret's triangle and periaqueductal gray matter

E. Medial longitudinal fasciculus (MLF) and central tegmental tract

Answer A

52. A congruous homonymous hemianopia with macular sparing is most often seen with occlusion of which of the following vessels?

A. Anterior choroidal artery

B. Posterior cerebral artery

C. Posterior choroidal artery

D. Posterior communicating artery

E. Recurrent artery of Heubner

Answer B

53. Following coronary artery bypass revascularization, a patient presents with simultanagnosia, optic ataxia, and apraxia of gaze. Which of the following is the most likely diagnosis?

A. Bilateral parietooccipital infarcts
B. Midbrain infarct
C. Paramedian thalamic infarcts
D. Bilateral orbitofrontal infarcts
E. Left mesiotemporal lobe infarct

Answer A

54. Which of the following is the most common cause of posterior cerebral artery (PCA) occlusion?

A. PCA dissection
B. Transtentorial herniation
C. Cardioembolism
D. Vertebrobasilar fibromuscular dysplasia
E. Antiphospholipid antibody syndrome

Answer C

55. Which of the following manifestations may increase the risk that patients may mistake the time of stroke onset?

A. Left hemiparesis
B. Ataxia
C. Internuclear ophthalmoplegia
D. Dissociated sensory loss
E. Left homonymous hemianopia

Answer E

56. Numbness, tingling, and painful hypersensitivity of the anterolateral thigh down to the upper patellar region are most characteristic of which of the following conditions?

A. L-4 radiculopathy
B. L-5 radiculopathy
C. Obturator neuropathy
D. Lateral femoral cutaneous neuropathy
E. Femoral neuropathy

Answer D

57. Which of the following is the most common entrapment neuropathy?

A. Posterior interosseus syndrome
B. Suprascapular nerve entrapment
C. Carpal tunnel syndrome

D. Deep ulnar nerve at the wrist

E. Radial nerve at the humerus

Answer C

58. A 60-year-old man has acute onset of severe back pain, numbness of both legs, and inability to void. On neurological examination, there is flaccid paraparesis and loss of pain and temperature sensation below the nipple line with sparing of touch, vibration, and position sense. Which of the following is the most likely diagnosis?

A. Syringomyelia

B. Spinal cord infarction

C. Viral myelitis

D. Spinal cord meningioma

E. Subacute combined degeneration (B_{12} deficiency)

Answer B

59. Heterochromia of the iris in a patient with a Horner's syndrome is indicative of which of the following:

A. Preganglionic lesion

B. Lesion occurrence before 2 years of age

C. Postganglionic lesion

D. Raeder paratrigeminal syndrome

E. Pancoast tumor

Answer B

60. Which of the following clinical features distinguishes fulminant hepatic failure from chronic portosystemic encephalopathy?

A. Tremor

B. Asterixis

C. Cerebral edema

D. Agitation

E. Confusion

Answer C

61. A 30-year-old man with Guillain-Barré syndrome should be intubated when the forced vital capacity drops below how many milliliters per kilogram?

A. 5

B. 40

C. 30

D. 15

E. 50

Answer D

62. Which of the following is the most likely diagnosis in a 30-year-old woman with new-onset bilateral asynchronus trigeminal neuralgia?

A. Syringobulbia
B. Basilar artery aneurysm
C. Brainstem glioma
D. Multiple sclerosis
E. Nasopharyngeal carcinoma

Answer D

63. Which of the following clinical features *excludes* the diagnosis of idiopathic trigeminal neuralgia?
    A. Mandibular trigeminal distribution
    B. Normal facial sensation
    C. Age group 60 to 70 years
    D. Right-sided predominance
    E. Loss of corneal reflex

    Answer E

64. The sudden onset of vertigo while trying to sit up suddenly, associated with rotatory nystagmus beating toward the downmost ear, with latency and limited duration is characteristic of which of the following disorders?
    A. Otosclerosis
    B. Ménière's disease
    C. Acoustic neuroma
    D. Benign paroxysmal positional vertigo
    E. Vertebrobasilar ischemia

    Answer D

65. Episodic vertigo, fluctuating hearing loss, tinnitus, and aural fullness are characteristic of which of the following disorders?
    A. Otosclerosis
    B. Ménière's disease
    C. Acoustic neuroma
    D. Benign paroxysmal positional vertigo
    E. Vertebrobasilar ischemia

    Answer B

66. Which of the following stroke syndromes is *not* at risk for intracranial hypertension?
    A. Main stem of middle cerebral artery occlusion
    B. Internal carotid artery occlusion
    C. Paramedian pontine infarction
    D. Aneurysmal subarachnoid hemorrhage
    E. Intracerebral hemorrhage

    Answer C

67. Which of the following parameters should be the primary goal of intracranial pressure (ICP) management in a monitored patient with an acute stroke?

A. ICP < 20 mm H_2O; cerebral perfusion pressure > 70 mm Hg
B. ICP < 50 mm H_2O; cerebral perfusion pressure > 100 mm Hg
C. ICP < 80 mm H_2O; cerebral perfusion pressure > 100 mm Hg
D. ICP < 70 mm H_2O; cerebral perfusion pressure > 20 mm Hg
E. ICP < 100 mm H_2O; cerebral perfusion pressure > 30 mm Hg
Answer A

68. Administration of mannitol for elevated intracranial pressure in a monitored patient should aim for which of the following serum osmolality values (mOsm)?

A. <250
B. <280
C. <300
D. <320
E. <350
Answer D

69. Which of the following medications should be started on arrival in patients with aneurysmal subarachnoid hemorrhage?

A. Nifedipine
B. Nimodipine
C. Labetalol
D. Nitroglycerin
E. Sodium nitroprusside
Answer B

70. Arterial hypotension during the first hours after thrombolysis for acute ischemic stroke should raise the concern for which of the following diagnoses?

A. SIADH
B. Central salt-wasting syndrome
C. Dehydration
D. Hemopericardium and cardiac tamponade
E. Pulmonary embolus
Answer D

71. Which of the following is the most common cause of spontaneous subarachnoid hemorrhage?

A. Ruptured cerebral arteriovenous malformation
B. Ruptured cerebral aneurysm
C. Coagulopathies
D. Vasculitides
E. Illicit drug use
Answer B

72. Which of the following is the most common location of saccular intracranial aneurysms?

A. Ophthalmic artery
B. Pericallosal artery
C. Anterior communicating artery
D. Basilar apex
E. Origin of posterior inferior cerebellar artery

Answer C

73. A 50-year-old man presents with complaints of fatigue and subjective weakness. Symptoms have been present for approximately 4 months. On examination, there is no atrophy or fasciculations and muscle strength testing is grossly normal. The patient has been a farmer for 30 years, drinks two beers a day, and has smoked one and a half packs of cigarettes per day for 35 years. Which of the following elements in his review of systems, if positive, would assist in focusing the diagnosis?

A. Low back pain
B. Intermittent right upper quadrant pain
C. Dry mouth
D. Remote exposure to pesticides
E. Tinnitus

Answer C

74. The above patient agrees to undergo EMG/NCS for further evaluation. Which of the following, if any, might confirm the clinical suspicion?

A. Low amplitudes in motor nerve conduction studies
B. Absent median sensory action potential
C. Incremental response seen in CMAP with high frequency (50 Hz) repetitive stimulation
D. A and C
E. None of the above

Answer C

75. A 65-year-old man presents with a 4-year history of progressive wasting and weakness of the bilateral upper extremities. There is no history of neck trauma or injury. The patient states that the symptoms began in his right arm and spread to involve the left about 1 year ago. There is no pain and no sensory complaint. The patient denies dysarthria and dysphagia. On examination, there is severe diffuse atrophy with weakness in muscles involving the median, ulnar, and radial nerves bilaterally. Laboratory data reveal normal ESR, TSH, Ca++, and elevated GM1 antibodies. The next step you would take with this patient is:

A. Repeat laboratory values in 6 months
B. Schedule EMG/NCS, cervical spine MRI, and brain MRI
C. Counsel the patient that he probably has ALS and nothing can be done
D. Discuss the risks and benefits of immunotherapy and plan for a course of either i.v. Ig or plasmapheresis
E. Recommend an intense course of physical therapy to build up arm strength

Answer D

76. A 6-month-old infant presents in the pediatric neurology clinic with failure to thrive. The infant is in the 1% range for weight, 50% for height and head circumference. The patient's mother reports that the infant has a difficult time feeding and a weak high-pitched cry, but is otherwise alert, responsive, and has a responsive smile. On examination, the patient cannot raise his head from a prone position and has decreased tone (floppy) in all extremities. An EMG performed earlier in the day revealed denervation with fibrillations and positive waves, with large rapid-firing motor units in all muscles evaluated. You discuss with the parents:

A. Brain MRI to evaluate for cerebral palsy
B. Fibroblasts for mucopolysaccharidoses
C. EEG for infantile spasms
D. Survival motor neuron gene testing for SMA
E. Muscle biopsy for nemaline rod myopathy

Answer D

77. A 35-year-old woman with genetically proven myotonic dystrophy presents to your clinic. Her chief complaint is fatigue. She has not seen a physician in several years. She complains of bilateral foot drop and distal hand stiffness but denies any other problems. Social history: She does not smoke or drink. She finished high school at 19 and took one semester of college work. She is recently married. In her family history, she reports that her father wears braces and uses CPAP at night. You recommend for the patient:

A. No need to worry, that everything appears fine.
B. Many myotonics are fatigued and she should "take it slow."
C. Baseline EKG, overnight polysomnography, and genetic counseling
D. MRI of the brain, EEG, and respiratory therapy
E. As a patient with myotonic dystrophy, she has decreased mental capacity and should appoint a power of attorney

Answer C

78. Which of the following angiopathies is caused by mutations in the notch 3 gene?

A. Fabry disease
B. CADASIL
C. Moyamoya
D. Susac syndrome
E. Fibromuscular dysplasia

Answer B

79. A 45-year-old man is unable to flex the distal phalanx of the thumb and index finger. There is no sensory loss. Which of the following is the most likely diagnosis?

A. Carpal tunnel syndrome
B. Posterior cord brachial plexopathy

C. Anterior interosseus syndrome

D. Radial neuropathy at the spiral groove

E. C-6 radiculopathy

Answer C

80. Which of the following is the most common location of ulnar nerve compression?

A. Axilla

B. Arm

C. Elbow

D. Wrist

E. Palm

Answer C

81. Following a bout of alcoholic intoxication, a 25-year-old man developed weakness of right wrist and finger extension and right brachioradialis, with preservation of triceps and deltoid function. Which of the following is the most likely diagnosis?

A. Posterior interosseus syndrome

B. Radial neuropathy at the spiral groove

C. Posterior cord brachial plexopathy

D. Radial sensory neuropathy

E. C-8 radiculopathy

Answer B

82. Following a weekend of archery competition, a 35-year-old woman complains of difficulty combing her hair. Examination shows winging of the medial border of the scapula. Which of the following nerves is most likely affected?

A. Axillary

B. Suprascapular

C. Spinal accessory

D. Long thoracic

E. Musculocutaneous

Answer D

83. Which of the following is *not* a feature of a common peroneal neuropathy?

A. Foot drop

B. Weakness of ankle dorsiflexion

C. Weakness of toe dorsiflexion

D. Weakness of ankle eversion

E. Weakness of plantar flexion

Answer E

84. The spinal accessory nerve exits the cranium through which of the following anatomical structures?

A. Hypoglossal canal
B. Jugular foramen
C. Stylomastoid foramen
D. Foramen lacerum
E. Foramen rotundum

Answer B

85. An 18-month-old child presented with macrocrania. CT scan demonstrated cystic dilatation of the fourth ventricle, cerebellar vermian dysgenesis, and hydrocephalus. Which of the following is the most likely diagnosis?

A. Chiari I malformation
B. Aqueductal stenosis
C. Joubert syndrome
D. Alexander disease
E. Dandy-Walker malformation

Answer E

86. Which of the following dementias have parietotemporal hypometabolism with sparing of the occipital cortex on FDG PET scans?

A. Dementia with Lewy bodies
B. Alzheimer disease
C. Dementia associated with Parkinson's disease
D. Huntington disease
E. Corticobasal degeneration

Answer B

87. Which of the following is the treatment of choice in patients with disabling upper limb poststroke spasticity?

A. Clonidine
B. Benzodiazepines
C. Botulinum toxin A
D. Phenytoin
E. Phenobarbital

Answer C

88. Which risk factor is most prevalent in patients with ischemic stroke?

A. Cigarette smoking
B. Diabetes mellitus
C. Hyperlipidemia
D. Hypertension
E. Prior transient ischemic attacks

Answer D

89. Which of the following symptomatic patients with hemispheric ischemia would benefit most from carotid endarterectomy?

A. Stenosis of 70% to 99% (not near occlusion)
B. Stenosis of 50% to 69%
C. String sign (tight stenosis with distal vessel collapse)
D. Stenosis of 30% to 50%
E. Stenosis less than 30%

Answer A

90. Stroke associated with migraine most commonly involves which of the following arterial territories?

A. Anterior choroidal
B. Anterior cerebral artery
C. Posterior cerebral artery
D. Middle cerebral artery
E. Ophthalmic artery

Answer C

91. Which of the following is the most common cause of iatrogenic accessory nerve palsy?

A. Posterior cervical lymph node dissection
B. Catheter cerebral angiography through a brachial approach
C. Tracheostomy
D. Reduction of shoulder subluxation
E. Lumbar puncture

Answer A

92. Which of the following is a potential risk of ventriculostomy in the treatment of patients presenting with hydrocephalus and cerebellar infarction?

A. Central herniation
B. Uncal herniation
C. Upward herniation
D. Transfalxine herniation
E. Kernohan notch syndrome

Answer C

93. Following carotid endarterectomy for treatment of symptomatic 90% stenosis of the right internal carotid artery, a 70-year-old hypertensive man experienced atypical migrainous phenomena, transient focal seizure activity, and a right hemispheric hematoma. Which of the following conditions most likely explains this postoperative complication?

A. Carotid dissection
B. Perioperative hypotension
C. Rupture of undiagnosed intacranial aneurysm
D. Hyperperfusion syndrome
E. Cerebral amyloid angiopathy

Answer D

94. Which of the following is the most common cause of ischemic stroke?

A. Atherothrombosis
B. Cervicocephalic arterial dissection
C. Vasculitis
D. Prothrombotic state
E. Cervicocephalic fibromuscular dysplasia

Answer A

95. Most deaths after first-ever stroke are due to which of the following conditions?

A. Pneumonia
B. Urosepsis
C. Renal failure
D. Cardiovascular event and recurrent stroke
E. SIADH

Answer D

96. Which of the following anatomical structures is responsible for most CSF formation?

A. Pineal gland
B. Lamina terminalis
C. Arachnoid granulations
D. Choroid plexus
E. Obex

Answer D

97. Which of the following anatomical structures is most responsible for CSF resorption?

A. Pineal gland
B. Lamina teminalis
C. Arachnoid granulations
D. Choroid plexus
E. Obex

Answer C

98. Febrile status epilepticus is the major cause of status epilepticus in which of the following age groups?

A. Less than 6 months
B. 1 to 2 years
C. 3 to 5 years
D. 6 to 8 years
E. 9 to 12 years

Answer B

99. In the acute management of seizures, which of the following drugs has the most favorable absorption after IM administration?

A. Lorazepam
B. Diazepam
C. Clonazepam
D. Midazolam
E. Paraldehyde

Answer D

100. After i.v. administration, which of the following drugs has the shortest time to peak brain concentration?

A. Lorazepam
B. Diazepam
C. Clonazepam
D. Phenytoin
E. Phenobarbital

Answer B

101. When administered as an i.v. loading dose, which of the following drugs has the lowest potential for respiratory depression?

A. Lorazepam
B. Diazepam
C. Clonazepam
D. Phenytoin
E. Phenobarbital

Answer D

102. A 65-year-old woman is brought to the emergency room following a fall down the stairs. On examination, she opens her eyes to voice. She does not follow commands but localizes to noxious stimulus and cannot carry on a conversation with one-word appropriate answers. Her Glasgow coma scale score is:

A. 5
B. Less than 8
C. 11
D. 14
E. 15

Answer C

103. Which of the following is *not* a paraclinical test used in the diagnosis of brain death?

A. Cerebral angiography
B. Nuclear medicine blood flow study
C. EEG
D. Transcranial Doppler ultrasound
E. MRI and/or MRA of the brain

Answer E

104. Which of these clinical features is *not* a significant determinant in determining the prognosis of a patient with an intracerebral hemorrhage?

A. Etiology of the hemorrhage
B. Patient age
C. Hematoma volume
D. Glasgow coma scale
E. Intraventricular extension

Answer A

105. In a 40-year-old patient with status epilepticus who continues to seize after receiving the maximum dose of intravenous lorazepam and a maximal loading dose of phenytoin (or the equivalent in fosphenytoin), the current preferred next step would be:

A. Give more lorazepam
B. Treat with a loading dose of carbamazepine
C. Give an additional 20 mg per kg loading dose of phenytoin
D. Treat with a propofol or midazolam drip
E. Confirm diagnosis by EEG

Answer D

106. Which of the following agents is *not* an inhibitor of acetylcholinesterase (AChE)?

A. Tacrine
B. Donepezil
C. Rivastigmine
D. Galantamine
E. Selegiline

Answer E

107. Early parkinsonian features, visual hallucinations, and fluctuations in cognitive function are most characteristic of which of the following dementias?

A. Pick disease
B. Alzheimer disease
C. Dementia with Lewy bodies
D. Hydrocephalic dementia
E. Vascular dementia

Answer C

108. Which of the following agents has been associated with an increased risk of stroke?

A. Quetiapine (Seroquel)
B. Olanzapine (Zyprexa)
C. Haloperidol (Haldol)
D. Risperidone (Risperdal)
E. Buspirone (BuSpar)

Answer B

109. Which of the following brain regions is most severely affected by the presence of neurofibrillary tangles in patients with Alzheimer dementia?

A. Primary motor cortex
B. Visual cortex
C. Primary sensory cortex
D. Entorhinal cortex and hippocampus
E. Anterior nuclei of the thalamus

Answer D

110. Diagnosis of Alzheimer disease is made by which of the following?

A. Tau protein in CSF
B. Genotyping for apolipoprotein
C. EEG
D. Single photon emission computerized tomography (SPECT) of the brain
E. Clinical criteria

Answer E

111. Which of the following is the most common clinical form of multiple sclerosis?

A. Relapsing-remitting
B. Primary progressive
C. Devic's disease (neuromyelitis optica)
D. Baló's concentric sclerosis
E. Acute fulminant form (Marburg's variant)

Answer A

112. A 30-year-old woman has a 3-day history of right orbital pain associated with eye movements and loss of vision of the right eye. On examination, visual acuity is 20/50 on the OD and 20/20 on the OS. There is red desaturation on the right eye, a right cecocentral scotoma, and a right relative afferent pupillary defect. Which of the following is the most likely diagnosis?

A. Central retinal artery occlusion
B. Anterior ischemic optic neuropathy
C. Optic neuritis
D. Posterior ischemic optic neuropathy
E. Cilioretinal artery occlusion

Answer C

113. Which of the following is the site of origin of the sympathetic pathway to the pupil?

A. Hypothalamus
B. Edinger-Westphal nucleus in the midbrain
C. Pontine paramedian reticular formation
D. Medial longitudinal fasciculus
E. Nucleus accumbens

Answer A

114. Which of the following is the site of origin of the parasympathetic pathway to the pupil?

A. Hypothalamus
B. Edinger-Westphal nucleus in the midbrain
C. Paramedian pontine reticular formation
D. Medial longitudinal fasciculus
E. Nucleus accumbens

Answer B

115. Which of the following is the location of the anatomical structures regulating oxygenation and acid-base balance?

A. Frontoorbital
B. Mesiotemporal
C. Insula of Reil
D. Lower brainstem
E. Midbrain tectum

Answer D

116. Which of the following is the basic substance for cerebral metabolism?

A. Phosphorus
B. Calcium
C. Glucose
D. Magnesium
E. Sodium

Answer C

117. Which of the following interventions should be *avoided* in the early (less than 4 hours) management of a comatose patient?

A. 5% dextrose in water intravenous infusion
B. Placement of large-bore intravenous catheter
C. Oropharyngeal airway
D. Vasoactive substances
E. Gastric lavage

Answer A

118. Flexion of the upper arms against the chest, pronation and flexion of the wrists, and extension of the lower extremities is an indication of which of the following conditions?

A. Decorticate posturing
B. Decerebrate posturing
C. Catatonia
D. Tetanus
E. Strychnine poisoning

Answer A

119. Extension of the elbows, pronation and extension of the wrists, and extension of the lower extremities is an indication of which of the following conditions?

A. Decortication
B. Decerebration
C. Catatonia
D. Tetanus
E. Strychnine poisoning

Answer B

120. In a comatose patient, extension of the elbows, pronation and extension of the wrists, and extension of the lower extremities is most likely an indication of a lesion at which of the following anatomical locations?

A. Bilateral orbitofrontal
B. Bilateral thalamic
C. Midbrain/upper pons
D. Cerebellum
E. Bilateral mesiotemporal

Answer C

121. In a comatose patient, flexion of the arms against the chest, pronation and flexion of the wrists, and extension of the lower extremities is most likely an indication of a lesion at which of the following anatomical locations?

A. Cerebellum
B. Midbrain/upper pons
C. Cerebral hemispheres and diencephalon
D. Medulla oblongata
E. Cervicomedullary junction

Answer C

122. Which of the following reflexes is tested with the doll's eyes maneuver?

A. Oculovestibular
B. Ciliospinal
C. Cochleopalpebral
D. Oculocephalic
E. Corneomandibular

Answer D

123. Which of the following tests is done to evaluate the oculovestibular reflex?

A. Apnea
B. Caloric (ice water)
C. Dix-Hallpike
D. Brainstem auditory evoked potential
E. Electrooculography

Answer B

124. A 60-year-old woman complains of nocturnal leg paresthesias with an irresistible urge to move the legs. There is partial relief by activity. Which of the following disorders is most commonly associated with her condition?

A. Hyperthyroidism
B. Hypoglycemia
C. Zinc deficiency
D. Iron deficiency anemia
E. Hypocalcemia

Answer D

125. Which of the following agents used in the treatment of Parkinson's disease can precipitate sleepiness with sudden sleep episodes?

A. Amantadine
B. Dopamine receptor agonists
C. Selegiline
D. L-dopa
E. Artane

Answer B

126. Which of the following is the drug of first choice in the management of restless legs syndrome?

A. L-dopa
B. Benzodiazepines
C. Lamotrigine
D. Haloperidol
E. Pimozide

Answer A

127. Which of the following neurological disorders can be improved by liver transplantation?

A. Acute intermittent porphyria
B. Fabry disease
C. Wilson disease
D. Chorea acanthocytosis
E. Menkes disease

Answer C

128. Which of the following transplant patients are at greater risk of developing central pontine myelinolysis (CPM) perioperatively?

A. Kidney
B. Heart
C. Lung
D. Liver
E. Pancreas

Answer D

129. Cortical blindness in allograft transplant patients is most commonly the result of toxicity by which of the following agents?

A. Corticosteroids
B. Cyclosporine
C. Azathioprine
D. Imipenem
E. Mycophenolate

Answer B

130. A 50-year-old obese man complains of morning headaches, mild memory difficulties, and excessive daytime sleepiness. His bed partner reports loud snoring. Which of the following is the most likely diagnosis?

A. Narcolepsy
B. Parasomnia
C. Restless legs syndrome
D. Obstructive sleep apnea
E. REM sleep behavior disorder

Answer D

131. A 55-year-old executive complains of creeping, crawling sensations of the legs associated with irresistible movements of the extremities most severe at bedtime. Symptoms are present at rest and are occasionally relieved by stretching or rubbing. Which of the following is the most likely diagnosis?

A. Narcolepsy
B. Delayed sleep phase syndrome
C. Restless legs syndrome
D. Obstructive sleep apnea
E. REM sleep behavior disorder

Answer C

132. An 18-year-old college student complains of excessive daytime sleepiness and irresistible episodes of falling asleep during classes and while driving. Which of the following is the most appropriate ancillary diagnostic test?

A. CSF levels of orexin (hypocretin)
B. Nocturnal polysomnography and multiple sleep latency
C. Apnea-hypopnea index
D. HLA typing
E. Neuropsychological testing

Answer B

133. Which of the following short-lasting headache types responds to indomethacin?

A. Trigeminal neuralgia
B. Cluster headaches
C. Paroxysmal hemicrania

   D. Short-lasting unilateral neuralgiform headache attacks with conjunctival in-
     jection and tearing (SUNCT)
   E. Hypnic headaches

Answer C

134. Retroperitoneal fibrosis is a potential complication of which of the following
drugs used for the treatment of headaches?

   A. Topiramate
   B. Methysergide
   C. Divalproex sodium
   D. Diltiazem
   E. Sumatriptan

Answer B

135. Which of the following is *not* a characteristic clinical feature of cluster
headaches?

   A. Lacrimation
   B. Nasal congestion
   C. Rhinorrhea
   D. Mydriasis
   E. Sense of restlessness during headache

Answer D

136. Diffuse meningeal enhancement on gadolinium-enhanced MRI is most characteristic of which of the following headache types?

   A. Cluster
   B. Paroxysmal hemicrania
   C. Short-lasting unilateral neuralgiform headache attacks with conjunctival in-
     jection and tearing (SUNCT)
   D. Chronic daily headache
   E. Intracranial hypotension and low-pressure headache

Answer E

137. Which of the following interventions reduces the risk of postlumbar puncture
headache?

   A. Use of large-gauge needles
   B. Use of cutting-tip needles
   C. Warning about postlumbar puncture headache
   D. Replacing stylet
   E. Lying supine for 4 hours after procedure

Answer D

138. Which of the following is the most common cause of nontraumatic coma?

   A. Hypoxia-ischemia
   B. Cerebral infarction
   C. Hepatic encephalopathy

D. Hyponatremia

E. Brain mass lesions

Answer A

139. Which of the following clinical/paraclinical features is **not** a poor prognostic indicator in patients with nontraumatic coma?

A. Glasgow coma scale (GCS) motor score of 6 at day 3

B. Absent pupillary response to light at day 3

C. Isoelectric EEG after 1 week

D. Bilateral absence of N20 after median nerve stimulation after 1 week

E. Burst-suppression EEG after 1 week

Answer A

140. Which of the following clinical manifestations is among the earliest clinical findings in children with neurofibromatosis type 1?

A. Café-au-lait spots

B. Axillary and inguinal freckles

C. Lisch nodules

D. Plexiform neurofibromas

E. Scoliosis

Answer A

141. Which of the following conditions may cause irreversible spinal cord damage in patients with Down syndrome?

A. Dural ectasias

B. Atlantoaxial instability

C. Spinal cord schwannomas

D. Spinal cord meningiomas

E. Subacute combined degeneration

Answer A

142. Which of the following tumors is most commonly seen in patients with tuberous sclerosis complex?

A. Meningioma

B. Optic nerve glioma

C. Subependymal giant cell astrocytoma

D. Plexiform neurofibroma

E. Hemangioblastoma

Answer C

143. CNS hemangioblastomas in patients with Von Hippel-Lindau disease are typically located in which of the following anatomical regions?

A. Thalamus

B. Optic chiasm

C. Midbrain

D. Occipital lobes

E. Cerebellum

Answer E

144. Which of the following features best characterizes cluster headaches?

A. Headaches lasting 1 or 2 days and recurring every 1 to 2 weeks in a 20-year-old woman

B. Bilateral moderately severe headaches in a 60-year-old man

C. Unilateral and severe headaches lasting minutes to a few hours, associated with rhinorrhea, ipsilateral miosis, and eyelid ptosis

D. Sudden onset of severe headaches with neck stiffness

E. Lingering orthostatic headaches

Answer C

145. Intracranial pain-sensitive structures include all of the following *except:*

A. Dura mater

B. Large cerebral vessels

C. Pial vessels

D. Brain parenchyma

E. Large venous sinuses

Answer D

146. Pain-producing intracranial structures are innervated by which of the following cranial nerves?

A. III

B. V

C. VII

D. IX

E. X

Answer B

147. Which of the following features best characterizes the mechanism of action of triptans?

A. Selective 5-HT1 agonists

B. Cyclooxygenase (COX) 1 inhibitors

C. Serotonin antagonists

D. Reversible monoamine oxidase inhibitors (MAOI)

E. Endothelin antagonists

Answer A

148. Which of the following is the most common emotional response after stroke?

A. Mania

B. Agitation

C. Emotional lability

D. Depression
E. Anxiety

Answer D

149. Of the following, which is the major cause of death for American women?

A. Multiple sclerosis
B. Stroke
C. Myasthenia gravis
D. Epilepsy
E. Parkinson's disease

Answer B

150. Which of the following is the most common adverse effect at the onset of therapy with IFN-β-1A for treatment of multiple sclerosis?

A. Headaches
B. Flulike symptoms
C. Seizures
D. Vomiting
E. Myositis

Answer B

151. Which of the following clinical features increases the risk of dying in patients with acute bacterial meningitis?

A. Fever
B. Arterial hypotension
C. Altered mental state
D. Community-acquired meningitis
E. Lack of neck stiffness

Answer B

152. A 40-year-old man developed burning right-sided otalgia, followed by periauricular paresthesias, vertigo, and rapidly developing right-sided peripheral facial weakness associated with vesicles in the ipsilateral ear. Which of the following ganglia is involved?

A. Superior cervical
B. Sphenopalatine
C. Geniculate
D. Gasserian
E. Nodose

Answer C

153. Which of the following cranial nerves is most commonly involved in patients with Lyme disease?

A. II
B. VII

C. III
D. XII
E. V

Answer B

154. Which of the following organisms is the most common etiologic agent of acute bacterial meningitis in adults (18 to 50 years of age) in the United States?

A. *Haemophilus influenzae*
B. *Listeria monocytogenes*
C. *N. meningitidis*
D. *Streptococcus agalactiae* (group B *streptococcus*)
E. *S. pneumoniae*

Answer E

155. Which of the following is the major cause of the aseptic meningitis syndrome?

A. Nonsteroidal antiinflammatory drugs (NSAIDs)
B. Antibiotics
C. i.v. Ig
D. Viruses
E. Parasites

Answer D

156. Which of the following is responsible for tetanus?

A. Tetanospasmin
B. Tetanolysin
C. Tetrodotoxin
D. Exotoxin of *Clostridium botulinum*
E. Toxin-producing dinoflagellates

Answer A

157. Which of the following dermatomes is most commonly affected by herpes zoster?

A. Trigeminal nerve
B. Cervical
C. Thoracic
D. Lumbar
E. Sacral

Answer C

158. Herpetic vesicles on the tip or side of the nose (Hutchinson sign) indicate involvement of which the following nerves?

A. Frontal nerve
B. Nasociliary nerve
C. Lacrimal nerve

D. Maxillary division of the trigeminal nerve
E. Mandibular division of the trigeminal nerve

Answer B

159. Capsaicin is a chemical that depletes which of the following transmitters?

A. Serotonin
B. Dopamine
C. Norepinephrine
D. Substance P
E. Glutamate

Answer D

160. Which of the following is *not* a typical feature of normal pressure hydrocephalus (NPH)?

A. Urinary incontinence
B. Memory impairment
C. Papilledema
D. Slowness of thought
E. Short-stepped and broad-based gait

Answer C

161. Which of the following clinical features is usually the first symptom in patients with normal pressure hydrocephalus (NPH)?

A. Gait disturbance
B. Dementia
C. Urinary incontinence
D. Seizures
E. Fecal incontinence

Answer A

162. Which of the following drugs decreases CSF production by the choroid plexus?

A. Hydrochlorothiazide
B. Indapamide
C. Triamterene
D. Acetazolamide
E. Nimodipine

Answer D

163. Which of the following organisms is most likely to cause meningitis as a complication of a neurosurgical procedure?

A. *L. monocytogenes*
B. *Staphylococcus aureus* and coagulase-negative staphylococci
C. *S. pneumoniae*

D. *N. meningitides*

E. *H. influenzae* Type b

Answer B

164. Which of the following organisms is the most common cause of acute sporadic encephalitis?

A. La Crosse virus

B. Epstein-Barr virus (EBV)

C. Varicella-zoster virus

D. HSV-1

E. Enteroviruses

Answer D

165. Which of the following organisms is the most common cause of viral meningitis?

A. La Crosse virus

B. Epstein-Barr virus (EBV)

C. Varicella-zoster virus

D. HSV-1

E. Enterovirus

Answer E

166. Which of the following viral infections in the first 12 weeks of pregnancy is a cause of intracranial calcifications, microcephaly, cataracts, sensorineural hearing loss, cardiac defects, and hepatosplenomegaly?

A. Rubella

B. Measles

C. Lymphocytic choriomeningitis

D. HSV-1

E. Hepatitis C

Answer A

167. Which of the following ischemic cerebrovascular disorders is less commonly associated with headaches?

A. Basilar artery occlusion

B. Stem of middle cerebral artery occlusion

C. Lacunar infarct

D. Internal carotid artery occlusion

E. Posterior cerebral artery occlusion

Answer C

168. Central nervous system myelin is produced by which of the following cells?

A. Microglia

B. Oligodendrocyte

C. Astrocyte

D. Purkinje

E. Schwann

Answer B

169. Which of the following disorders is the most common cause of tremor at rest?

A. Parkinson's disease

B. Essential tremor

C. Alcohol intoxication

D. Wilson's disease

E. Peripheral neuropathy

Answer A

170. Which of the following inclusions in the substantia nigra is characteristic of Parkinson's disease?

A. Negri bodies

B. Hirano bodies

C. Lyssa bodies

D. Lewy bodies

E. Bunina bodies

Answer D

171. A 55-year-old man is found at autopsy to have focal hemorrhagic lesions of the inferior part of the corpus callosum and dorsolateral quadrants of the rostral brainstem adjacent to the superior cerebellar peduncle, associated with diffuse axonal damage. Which of the following disorders is the most likely diagnosis?

A. Anoxic encephalopathy

B. Carbon monoxide intoxication

C. Diffuse axonal injury

D. Fat embolism

E. Hemorrhagic leukoencephalitis

Answer C

172. Which of the following features is *not* characteristic of cytomegalovirus polyradiculopathy in HIV disease?

A. Subacute lower back pain

B. Areflexic paraparesis

C. Distal sensory loss

D. Urinary difficulties

E. Normal CSF

Answer E

173. Which of the following is the most common peripheral nerve manifestation in seroconversion-related neuropathies in HIV disease?

A. Facial nerve palsy

B. Syphilitic polyradiculopathy

C. Hepatitis C infection–related neuropathy
D. Cytomegalovirus-related polyradiculpathy
E. Motor neuron disease syndrome

Answer A

174. Which of the following aphasias is most commonly seen in the early stages of Alzheimer disease?

A. Broca
B. Wernicke
C. Anomic
D. Conduction
E. Transcortical sensory

Answer C

175. Which of the following organisms is most commonly associated with subdural effusions in infants?

A. *S. pneumoniae*
B. *N. meningitides*
C. *L. monocytogenes*
D. *H. influenzae* Type b
E. *S. agalactiae*

Answer D

176. Which of the following intracranial tumors is most commonly associated with neurofibromatosis type 2?

A. Acoustic neuromas (vestibular schwannomas)
B. Cerebellar hemangioblastomas
C. Subependymal giant cell astrocytomas
D. Colloid cysts of the third ventricle
E. Medulloblastomas

Answer A

177. Which of the following drugs is most effective in the treatment of trigeminal neuralgia associated with multiple sclerosis?

A. Topiramate
B. Misoprostol
C. Cannabis
D. Levetiracetam
E. Primidone

Answer B

178. Which of the following clinical features of patients with aneurysmal subarachnoid hemorrhage (SAH) increases the risk of misdiagnosis?

A. Right-sided aneurysms
B. Hunt-Hess grade I or II

C. Left-sided aneurysms
D. Aneurysm size 7 to 10 mm
E. Lack of prior history of headaches

Answer B

179. For any given duration of ischemia following cardiac arrest, which of the following CNS regions is most vulnerable?

A. Thalamus
B. Midbrain
C. Pons
D. Cerebral cortex
E. Spinal cord

Answer D

180. Which of the following disorders is associated with elevation of myelin basic protein in the CSF?

A. Stroke
B. Multiple sclerosis
C. Head injury
D. Intracranial tumors
E. All of the above

Answer E

181. What percentage of the population harbors an unruptured intracranial aneurysm?

A. 30
B. 25
C. 3
D. 15
E. 20

Answer C

182. Which of the following unruptured intracranial aneurysms have the lowest annualized risk of subarachnoid hemorrhage (SAH)?

A. Anterior circulation aneurysms less than 7 mm
B. Basilar artery aneurysms
C. Giant aneurysms
D. Aneurysms less than 10 mm with associated SAH from another aneurysm
E. MCA aneurysms

Answer A

183. Which of the following best characterizes cerebral edema due to stroke?

A. Response to corticosteroid therapy
B. Response to barbiturates
C. Peak occurrence 3 to 5 days after stroke

D. Less severe among younger patients with MCA stem occlusion

E. Response to NMDA receptor antagonists

Answer C

184. What is the 30-day mortality rate for aneurysmal subarachnoid hemorrhage (SAH)?

A. 5%

B. 45%

C. 2%

D. 10%

E. 15%

Answer B

185. Which of the following is the most powerful predictor of 30-day mortality following aneurysmal subarachnoid hemorrhage (SAH)?

A. Anterior circulation aneurysms

B. Cerebral vasosopasm

C. Volume of initial SAH

D. Hunt-Hess grade I or II

E. Family history of aneurysmal SAH

Answer C

186. Which of the following electrolyte/metabolic abnormality causes a depression of the muscle stretch reflexes?

A. Hypoglycemia

B. Hypermagnesemia

C. Hyperkalemia

D. Hyponatremia

E. Hypocalcemia

Answer B

187. Which of the following is best avoided in the management of aneurysmal subarachnoid hemorrhage in the ICU?

A. Induced hypertension

B. Hypothermia

C. Nimodipine

D. Hypovolemia

E. Hyperventilation

Answer D

188. Which of the following best predicts the occurrence of cerebral vasospasm in patients with aneurysmal subarachnoid hemorrhage?

A. Male gender

B. Hunt-Hess grade I or II

C. Hyperglycemia

D. Volume of SAH on initial CT

E. Lack of intraventricular hemorrhage

Answer D

189. Which of the following movement disorders is most commonly associated with the chronic administration of opioids?

A. Tics

B. Chorea

C. Parkinsonism

D. Myoclonus

E. Athetosis

Answer D

190. Which of the following is the most commonly affected cranial nerve in sarcoidosis?

A. III

B. VII

C. II

D. VIII

E. V

Answer B

191. Which of the following is a major side effect of mitoxantrone?

A. Depression

B. Flulike symptoms

C. Cardiomyopathy

D. Neuropathy

E. Injection-site reactions

Answer C

192. Which of the following arthropathies may cause a cauda equina syndrome?

A. Osteoarthritis

B. Rheumatoid arthritis

C. Gout

D. Ankylosing spondylitis

E. Pseudogout

Answer D

193. Which of the following electrophysiologic testing is especially helpful in detecting clinically silent lesions in patients with multiple sclerosis?

A. Visual evoked potentials

B. Brainstem auditory evoked potentials

C. Electronystagmogram

D. Electroretinogram

E. EEG

Answer A

194. Among all brain tumors, which of the following is the most common?

A. Oligodendroglioma
B. Glioblastoma multiforme
C. Ependymoma
D. Meningioma
E. Metastases

Answer E

195. Which of the following is the most common primary brain tumor?

A. Oligodendroglioma
B. Glioblastoma multiforme
C. Ependymoma
D. Meningioma
E. Primary CNS lymphoma

Answer B

196. A 50-year-old woman has an intracranial meningioma. Examination shows anosmia, ipsilateral optic atrophy, and contralateral papilledema. Which of the following is the location of the tumor?

A. Cavernous sinus
B. Cerebellopontine angle
C. Olfactory groove
D. Sphenoid wing
E. Subfrontal

Answer C

197. Which of the following is the most common complication of medulloblastoma?

A. Deafness
B. Facial nerve palsy
C. Hydrocephalus
D. Third cranial nerve palsy
E. Seizures

Answer C

198. In patients with childhood epileptic encephalopathy (Lennox-Gastaut syndrome), corpus callosotomy is effective in reducing which of the following type of seizures?

A. Axial tonic
B. Drop attacks
C. Atypical absences
D. Complex partial
E. Generalized tonic-clonic

Answer B

199. Which of the following is a major complication of rapid correction of hyperglycemia and hyperosmolality in a patient with type II diabetes and nonketotic hyperosmolar state (NKHS)?

A. Central pontine myelinolysis
B. Marchiafava-Bignami disease
C. Cerebral edema
D. Orthostatic hypotension
E. Hypothermia

Answer C

200. Which of the following choreatic disorders is associated with an axonal sensorimotor polyneuropathy with amyotrophy?

A. Sydenham
B. Huntington
C. Wilson
D. Neuroacanthocytosis
E. Paroxysmal kinesiogenic dyskinesia

Answer D

201. Which of the following cardiac disorders is a complication of the vein of Galen malformation?

A. Complete heart block
B. Prolonged QT interval
C. High output cardiac failure
D. Restrictive cardiomyopathy
E. Torsades de pointes

Answer C

202. A 15-year-old adolescent boy has progressive muscle wasting and weakness in a scapulohumeroperoneal distribution, elbow and neck contractures, and cardiac conduction defects. Which of the following is the most likely diagnosis?

A. Duchenne muscular dystrophy
B. Becker muscular dystrophy
C. Myotonic dystrophy
D. Emery-Dreifuss muscular dystrophy
E. Limb girdle muscular dystrophy

Answer D

203. Which of the following syndromes causing mental retardation is associated with a trinucleotide repeat expansion?

A. Down
B. Fragile X
C. Cri-du-chat

D. Prader-Willi

E. Angelman

Answer B

204. Dystonia with diurnal variation (worse later in the day) in a 10-year-old girl is best treated with which of the following drugs?

A. Carbamazepine

B. Valproate

C. Lamotrigine

D. Levodopa

E. Mestinon

Answer D

205. Which of the following peroxisomal disorders is associated with a typical posterior white matter involvement on MRI?

A. Adrenoleukodystrophy

B. Zellweger syndrome

C. Refsum's disease

D. Hyperoxaluria type 1

E. Glutaryl CoA oxidase deficiency

Answer A

206. Which of the following autonomic disturbances in alcoholic neuropathy is due to sympathetic dysfunction?

A. Dysphagia

B. Dysphonia

C. Sleep apnea

D. Orthostatic hypotension

E. Depressed reflex heart response

Answer D

207. Central pontine myelinolysis may result from rapid correction of which of the following electrolyte disorders?

A. Hypomagnesemia

B. Hypophosphatemia

C. Hyponatremia

D. Hypocalcemia

E. Hypokalemia

Answer C

208. Which of the following is the most common cause of sudden worsening of spasticity in multiple sclerosis?

A. Cold showers

B. Sleep deprivation

C. Aerobic exercise

D. Urinary tract infection

E. Pain

Answer D

209. Which of the following is the most sensitive test for the diagnosis of multiple sclerosis?

A. MRI of brain

B. CT scan of brain

C. Visual evoked potentials

D. CSF analysis

E. Electronystagmogram

Answer A

210. Which of the following is the most common cause of vitamin B_{12} (cobalamin) deficiency?

A. Tropical sprue

B. Pernicious anemia

C. Blind loop syndrome

D. Methylmalonic aciduria

E. Whipple's disease

Answer B

211. Which of the following CNS areas is mostly affected by gross atrophy in Huntington's disease?

A. Cerebellar vermis

B. Pontine tegmentum

C. Caudate nucleus

D. Superficial layers of cerebral cortex

E. Thalamus

Answer C

212. Which of the following sensory modalities is interrupted by a syrinx?

A. Light touch

B. Vibration

C. Joint position sense

D. Pain and temperature

E. None of the above

Answer D

213. Which of the following sensory modalities is affected early in the course of subacute combined degeneration due to cobalamin (B_{12}) deficiency?

A. Light touch

B. Joint position and vibration

C. Pain
D. Temperature
E. None of the above

Answer B

214. A 10-year-old boy with mild kyphoscoliosis has progressive limb and gait ataxia. Examination shows distal weakness of the legs and feet and loss of position and vibration sense. Muscle stretch reflexes are absent in the legs. Plantar responses are extensor bilaterally. Which of the following is the most likely diagnosis?

A. Homocystinuria
B. Neuroacanthocytosis
C. Friedreich's ataxia
D. Chronic inflammatory demyelinating polyneuropathy
E. Refsum's disease

Answer C

215. Which of the following is the most common form of diabetic neuropathy?

A. Cranial neuropathy
B. Lumbosacral polyradiculopathy
C. Autonomic neuropathy
D. Distal sensorimotor polyneuropathy
E. Trunk mononeuropathy

Answer D

216. Which of the following is the most common location of a hypertensive intra-parenchymal hemorrhage?

A. Cerebellum
B. Lobar
C. Pons
D. Putamen
E. Thalamus

Answer D

217. Which of the following is a major cause of lobar hemorrhage in an elderly normotensive person?

A. Bleeding diathesis
B. Aspirin therapy
C. Ruptured cavernous malformations
D. Telangiectases
E. Cerebral amyloid angiopathy

Answer E

218. Which of the following is the most common focal opportunistic brain infection in patients with AIDS?

A. Cryptococcoma
B. Tuberculoma

C. Syphilitic gumma
D. Cerebral toxoplasmosis
E. *Nocardia* brain abscess

Answer D

219. Which of the following is the treatment of choice in patients with AIDS and single or multiple focal brain lesions?

A. Radiation therapy
B. Empiric trial of pyrimethamine, sulfadiazine, and folinic acid
C. Intravenous amphotericin B and fluconazole
D. High-dose intravenous dexamethasone
E. Intravenous ceftriaxone or penicillin

Answer B

220. Which of the following vessels is most commonly involved in patients with acute epidural hematoma?

A. Anterior ethmoidal artery
B. Middle meningeal artery
C. Transverse sinus
D. Sigmoid sinus
E. Superior sagittal sinus

Answer B

221. Chronic subdural hematoma is most commonly the result of rupture of which of the following vessels?

A. Anterior ethmoidal artery
B. Middle meningeal artery
C. Transverse sinus
D. Cortical bridging veins
E. Superior sagittal sinus

Answer D

222. Which of the following antiepileptic drugs may increase the risk of myoclonic seizures in patients with juvenile myoclonic epilepsy?

A. Valproic acid (Depakene)
B. Lamotrigine (Lamictal)
C. Topiramate (Topamax)
D. Carbamazepine (Tegretol)
E. Divalproex sodium (Depakote)

Answer D

223. Which of the following visual field deficits is most characteristic of chiasmal compression?

A. Bitemporal superior quadrantanopia
B. Bilateral central scotomas

C. Bilateral superior altitudinal defects
D. Bilateral inferior altitudinal defects
E. Bilateral enlargement of the blind spots

Answer A

224. Which of the following is the characteristic interictal EEG pattern in patients with infantile spasms (West syndrome)?

A. Burst suppression
B. Hypsarrhythmia
C. Unifocal or multifocal delta activity
D. Multifocal sharp waves
E. Positive rolandic sharp waves

Answer B

225. Which of the following is the treatment of choice for HSV-1 encephalitis?

A. Vidarabine
B. Acyclovir
C. Famciclovir
D. Didanosine
E. Zalcitabine

Answer B

226. Which of the following vitamins reduces the risk of neural tube defects in the general population?

A. Vitamin E
B. Cobalamin
C. Thiamine
D. Folic acid
E. Vitamin D

Answer D

227. Which of the following antiepileptic drugs may result in oral contraceptive failure?

A. Gabapentin
B. Carbamazepine
C. Valproic acid
D. Lamotrigine
E. Felbamate

Answer B

228. Which of the following paraneoplastic disorders is associated with anti–calcium channel antibodies (N and P/Q types)?

A. Sensory neuronopathy
B. Cerebellar degeneration

C. Lambert-Eaton myasthenic syndrome
D. Opsoclonus-myoclonus
E. Limbic encephalitis

Answer C

229. Which of the following primary brain tumors is more common in women with breast cancer?

A. Low-grade astrocytoma
B. Oligodendroglioma
C. Ependymoma
D. Primary CNS lymphoma
E. Meningioma

Answer E

230. Which of the following vitamin excess states results in sensory ataxia?

A. Vitamin A
B. Vitamin K
C. Cobalamin
D. Pyridoxine
E. Thiamine

Answer D

231. Which of the following drugs can cause a toxic myopathy with abnormal mitochondria resembling ragged red fibers?

A. Pentazocine
B. Glucocorticoids
C. Zidovudine (AZT)
D. Penicillamine
E. Lovastatin

Answer C

232. Which of the following microorganisms has been associated with the axonal form of Guillain-Barré syndrome?

A. *Karwinskia humboldtiana*
B. *Campylobacter jejuni*
C. *Citrobacter diversus*
D. *Pseudoallescheria*
E. *Cladosporium*

Answer B

233. Which of the following is an exclusion for the use of intravenous tPA in acute ischemic stroke?

A. Lacunar stroke
B. NIH stroke scale less than 8

C. Systolic blood pressure greater than 200 mm Hg
D. Platelet count less than 150,000
E. CT scan evidence of leukoaraiosis
Answer C

234. Which of the following is the most common involuntary movement disorder in metabolic encephalopathy?

A. Tremor
B. Chorea
C. Hemiballismus
D. Dystonia
E. Myoclonus
Answer E

235. Which of the following cranial nerves may be injured as a result of carotid endarterectomy?

A. III
B. VI
C. VII
D. XII
E. V
Answer D

For each disorder, select the most appropriate diagnosis/answer.

236. Abrupt onset, abrupt ending

A. Complex partial seizures
B. Absence seizures
C. Both
D. Neither
Answer B

237. Unawareness

A. Complex partial seizures
B. Absence seizures
C. Both
D. Neither
Answer C

238. Increased risk of neural tube defects

A. Valproate
B. Carbamazepine
C. Both
D. Neither
Answer C

239. Cerebral edema of metastatic brain disease

A. Cytotoxic
B. Vasogenic
C. Interstitial
D. Ischemic
E. Pyogenic

Answer B

240. Diabetes insipidus

A. Craniopharyngioma
B. Neurosarcoidosis
C. Both
D. Neither

Answer C

241. Paraneoplastic cerebellar degeneration

A. Anti-Yo antibodies
B. Anti-Hu antibodies
C. Both
D. Neither

Answer C

242. Hyperprolactinemia

A. Antipsychotics
B. Primary hypothyroidism
C. Both
D. Neither

Answer C

243. Pheochromocytoma

A. Neurofibromatosis
B. Von Hippel-Lindau disease
C. Both
D. Neither

Answer C

244. Mees lines

A. Arsenic toxicity
B. Thallium toxicity
C. Both
D. Neither

Answer C

245. Spasticity in multiple sclerosis

    A. Baclofen
    B. Tizanidine
    C. Both
    D. Neither

Answer C

246. Medulloblastoma

    A. Turcot syndrome (glioma poliposis syndrome)
    B. Von Hippel-Lindau disease
    C. Both
    D. Neither

Answer A

247. Autosomal dominant

    A. Huntington's disease
    B. Friedreich's ataxia
    C. Both
    D. Neither

Answer A

248. Autosomal recessive

    A. Huntington's disease
    B. Friedreich's ataxia
    C. Both
    D. Neither

Answer B

249. Trinucleotide repeat expansion

    A. Huntington's disease
    B. Friedreich's ataxia
    C. Both
    D. Neither

Answer C

250. Higher risk of Bell's palsy

    A. Diabetes mellitus
    B. Pregnancy
    C. Both
    D. Neither

Answer C

251. Tendon xanthomata

    A. Familial hypercholesterolemia
    B. Cerebrotendinous xanthomatosis

C. Both
D. Neither
Answer C

252. Physical complaints seen as intentional, voluntary, and consciously produced

A. Malingering
B. Conversion disorder
C. Both
D. Neither
Answer A

253. Alien limb phenomenon

A. Corticobasal degeneration
B. Callosal infarction
C. Both
D. Neither
Answer C

254. Most common adult-onset dystonias

A. Cervical dystonia
B. Blepharospasm
C. Both
D. Neither
Answer C

255. Response to low-doses of L-dopa

A. Myoclonic dystonia (DYT 11)
B. Paroxysmal kinesogenic dyskinesia (DTY 10)
C. Both
D. Neither
Answer D

256. Retinal hemorrhages

A. Optic neuritis
B. Anterior ischemic optic neuropathy
C. Both
D. Neither
Answer B

257. Compared to adults with optic neuritis, optic neuritis in children is more often

A. Bilateral
B. Parainfectious demyelinating
C. Both
D. Neither
Answer C

258. Idiopathic intracranial hypertension (pseudotumor cerebri)

A. Elevated CSF opening pressure above 180 mm water measured in lateral decubitus position

B. Elevated CSF opening pressure above 250 mm of water measured in lateral decubitus position

C. Both

D. Neither

Answer B

259. Conjunctival injection

A. Cluster headache

B. Trigeminal neuralgia

C. Both

D. Neither

Answer A

260. More common in women

A. Migraine headache

B. Chronic paroxysmal hemicrania

C. Both

D. Neither

Answer C